Albert Sims

The Common Use of Tobacco

Condemned by Physicians, Experience, Common Sense and the Bible

Albert Sims

The Common Use of Tobacco
Condemned by Physicians, Experience, Common Sense and the Bible

ISBN/EAN: 9783337092474

Printed in Europe, USA, Canada, Australia, Japan

Cover: Foto ©Lupo / pixelio.de

More available books at **www.hansebooks.com**

THE COMMON USE

OF

TOBACCO

Condemned by Physicians, Experience, Common Sense and the Bible.

By REV. A. SIMS.

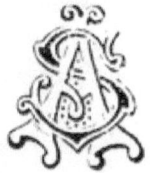

Prices: Cloth Covers, 50c.; Paper Covers, 30c.

———

REV. A. SIMS,
UXBRIDGE, ONTARIO, CANADA.

PREFACE.

SOME years ago we wrote and published a book, entitled "The Sin of Tobacco Smoking and Chewing," etc. We have reason to believe that, through the divine blessing, it accomplished some good. We are encouraged by the results to try a second edition. The work has been greatly enlarged and revised, and several new chapters have been added. The title has been changed to one which we think is more expressive of its contents. We assure the lover of the weed who may read these pages, that they have been written in the kindliest spirit, and with a sincere desire to benefit him, by pointing out to him the fearful injury tobacco does to his physical, mental and moral being. We, therefore, beg of him to give the arguments here brought forward a candid and careful perusal, believing that if they are read in this spirit, certain good will result.

THE AUTHOR.

CONTENTS.

CHAPTER I.   PAGE
The Uncleanness of Tobacco Habits   9

CHAPTER II.
The Enslaving Power of Tobacco, ... 14

CHAPTER III.
The Idolatry of Tobacco Habits 18

CHAPTER IV.
Tobacco and Hard Times 20

CHAPTER V.
Tobacco Injures the Mental Powers 23

CHAPTER VI.
Tobacco Leads to Insanity 29

CHAPTER VII.
Tobacco and Disease. 34

CHAPTER VIII.
Tobacco Users More Liable to Disease 63

CHAPTER IX.
Tobacco-Using Parents Injure their Offspring 69

CHAPTER X.
The Use of Tobacco a Curse to Boys and Young Men 76

CHAPTER XI.
Tobacco the Handmaid of Intemperance 81

CHAPTER XII.
The Common Use of Tobacco a Sin Against Society 86

CHAPTER XIII.
Does the Tobacco Habit Glorify God ? 91

CHAPTER XIV.
The Example of Smoking and Chewing Pernicious......... 94

CHAPTER XV.
Facts for Tobacco-Using Ministers.......... 96

CHAPTER XVI.
The Common Use of Tobacco a Direct Curse to the Soul .. 102

CHAPTER XVII.
The Time Wasted in the Indulgence of Tobacco 109

CHAPTER XVIII.
Tobacco a Destroyer of Property .... :...... 111

CHAPTER XIX.
Tobacco Impoverishes the Soil 112

CHAPTER XX.
Can a Christian Sell Tobacco?......... 116

CHAPTER XXI.
The Doubts of Tobacco Devotees 120

CHAPTER XXII.
Twelve Pleas Answered.... 122

CHAPTER XXIII.
Progress of the Anti-Tobacco Movement................... 134

CHAPTER XXIV.
Fifty-four Objections to Tobacco 139

CHAPTER XXV.
Christian Ladies vs. Tobacco 143

CHAPTER XXVI.
Miscellaneous Facts...................................... 150
Chronological Abstract of the Invasion of Tobacco........ 158
Smoking and Chewing—A Parody 160

CHAPTER XXVII.
The Infallible Cure 161

The Common Use of Tobacco.

CHAPTER I.

THE UNCLEANNESS OF TOBACCO HABITS.

"Let us cleanse ourselves from all filthiness of the flesh and spirit, perfecting holiness in the fear of God."

"If any man defile the temple of God, him shall God destroy; for the temple of God is holy, whose temple ye are."

THE central idea of the religion of Christ is purity; and it applies to the body as well as to the soul. Is it any wonder that God requires a pure temple to dwell in? Would we offer a dear friend, who came to see us, a filthy room to occupy? Nay; we would provide for his reception with the greatest care. How much more careful should we be to furnish a pure temple for the Holy Spirit to dwell in? We are to present "our bodies a living sacrifice," and to keep under the body; of course we include the passions, lusts, carnal affections—anything contrary to the principle of faith, or the law of love; anything that would, in any way, supplant the indwelling of the Divine Being. Now, how can a man be said to keep under the body, when at his leisure, he must partake of that which, to a considerable degree, clogs the brain with a breathed smoke, and pampers the affections of the flesh? The common use of tobacco is a most filthy habit to lungs, mouth and clothes; it is a perfect stench. It is not necessary to see a pipe in a man's mouth to know whether he is a smoker; he literally stinks as he goes about; his very breath is fetid and loathsome. How can such uncleanness be reconciled with the purity required by the Gospel of God? If cleanliness is a part of Christianity, and it undoubtedly is, to be filthy is to be wicked; yet the common use of tobacco is extremely filthy, and therefore sinful. Besides, God positively asserts in His Word, that he who dares to defile His temple shall be destroyed.

We do not expect anything better of horse-jockeys and debauchees, than that they should indulge in such filthy lusts of the flesh; but the children of God—the men and women who profess the holy religion of Christ—are expected to put away every unclean thing, and to abstain even from the appearance of evil. A Methodist exhorter and class-leader came up to a preacher one day, and, while tobacco spittle was running down from both corners of his mouth, he said: "I am going in for sanctification." The answer was: "Brother, begin right in your mouth."

A certain blacksmith used tobacco for about sixty years; he became convinced of the filthiness of his practice in the following manner: When working on hot iron there arose an odor very offensive, yes, almost unbearable. Its character was like tobacco spittle falling on a hot stove. The English language fails to express the feeling that a clean, sensitive, pure body has when it comes in contact with such fluid. This man could not bear this awful condition of things, and he wondered whence it came. It occurred to him that the cause was in himself. It was hot weather, and he was working hard and sweating freely, and drops of sweat fell quite often on the hot iron. To make the thing certain, he put a hoe into the forge, and when it was red hot, he took it out, and with his hand wiped the sweat from his face upon the hot hoe. And, O! whew what an odor ! Can it be that I am so filthy ? He was more than convinced, and resolved to abandon the habit forever.

Neither is filthiness of the flesh condemned only by the Christian ; for Mohammed, in harmony with Bible sentiments, anathematizes impurity. In his fifth commandment he says : " Keep thy body clean."

" Tobacco is a powerful agent in the removal of vermin from cattle. Farmers have applied it in decoction to calves, and not unfrequently it has occasioned death. It might be lawful to chew it when a man should find himself internally infested with vermin, until he shall have purged himself from such an engorgement, and it ought everywhere to be restricted to such a use : so that it should always be understood, when we see a man with a quid, or pipe, or cigar, stuck in the upper orifice of his body, that it is because he has become so internally verminized that he finds himself obliged to resort to this desperate measure, as his last effort to remove this awful calamity."— *Dr. Coles.*

" Dr. Lawson, late surgeon-general of the United States army, says he often observed that when the wolves and buzzards came upon the battle-fields to devour the slain, they would not disturb the bodies of those who had chewed or smoked tobacco until they had consumed all the others among them. And yet there are thousands of presumptuous young smokers and chewers who expect that refined young ladies will be willing to love and cherish all their lives what even buzzards will reject as nauseating and unwholesome."

Dr. Clarke quotes thus from a treatise written by Simon Paulli, physician to the King of Denmark : " Merchants frequently lay it in bog-houses, to the end that, becoming impregnated with the volatile salt of the excrements, it may be rendered brisker and stronger." Speaking for himself, Dr. Clarke says : " A dealer once acknowledged to me that he frequently sprinkled his rolls and leaf with stale urine to keep them moist and preserve the flavor. A friend of mine, whose curiosity led him to see tobacco-spinning, observed that the boys who opened out the dry plants had a vessel of urine by them, with which they moistened the leaves to prepare them for the spinner. Do the tobacco chewers know this, and yet continue in this most abominable and disgusting practice? Can any person think of the above with a *quid* in his mouth? Were this offensiveness confined to the users it would be bad enough, but it is not, but is a source of annoyance and discomfort to others as well."

Chester E. Pond, in his tract, entitled "A Tornado Among the Human Tobacco Shrubs," asks the following pertinent questions: "Why is it that men are always ashamed to smoke in the presence of the purest and best society? Why is it that those wishing to smoke sneak off to the dirtiest car on a train, or to the dirtiest room in a hotel? Why is it that boys, when wishing to learn the filthy habit, usually seek the vilest company, and then try to secrete themselves in some dingy garret, dirty alley, or disgusting outhouse? Simply because beastly habits seem most appropriate and are best enjoyed in beastly places. When all restraint is removed, and men are left free to enjoy their own hearts' love, they always feel most at home where their external surroundings correspond to their internal states."

Dr. Coles, says: "There are but three kinds of animals, which generally use tobacco: The rock goat of Africa—whose stench is so unsufferable that no other animal can approach it; the tobacco worm, whose intolerable visage gives to every beholder an involuntary shudder; and one other nondescript animal, whose tobacco frothings and

spittings defile his own visage, bespatter and bedaub everything within his reach ; who pollutes the atmosphere with
his nauseous fumigations, and whose Stygian breath seems
to denote approximation to some bottomless pit."

Dr. Welsh, of Yale College, says : " The tobacco user is
giving forth pestilential vapors from all the pores of his
skin ; he is the embodiment of perpetual miasma—a walking distillery of deadly essence." If your cat should use
the filthy weed, you would kill the unclean animal.

In 1492, as Columbus lay with his ships side by side at
the Island of Cuba, he sent two men, a " Caleb and
Joshua," to search the land and report what they might
see.   On their return, among other things, they said they
saw " the naked savages twist large leaves together, light
one end at the fire, and smoke like devils ! "   Smokers
should bear in mind their pedigree ! Barbarous ! Sensual !
Devilish !

" In the house of God, where, of all other places, decency
and cleanliness should be observed, it is appalling to notice
the repulsive and abominably filthy state of many of the
pews, rendered so by the spitting habits of those who
smoke or chew tobacco.   Churches are most scandalously
used by the tobacco chewers who frequent them ; and
kneeling before the Great Jehovah, which is so becoming
when sinners approach their Maker in prayer, is rendered
impossible in many seats for ladies, because of the large
quantity of tobacco saliva which is ejected in all directions."—*Dr. A. Clarke.*

A snuff-taker of twenty-eight years' standing, determined to give up the habit, after reading the following
sentence : " Next to dying an unpardoned transgressor, I
should shrink from the idea of being laid in my coffin with
my nostrils charged with snuff."

A Baptist minister had used tobacco some twenty-five or thirty years, and although he always felt morally restrained from further indulgence, yet the flesh (?) was too weak, until the flesh began to suffer for it in the shape of a large tumor under the arm. Imagine this reverend gentleman's surprise, and fright, too, when the surgeon opened the tumor and found it nothing more or less than a tobacco tumor !! Its contents smelled as strongly of tobacco as any old pipe ! Whew ! what a stench !

What a striking illustration are the above incidents of these oft-forgotten words : "Be not deceived ; God is not mocked : for whatsoever a man soweth, that shall he also reap. For he that soweth to his flesh, shall of the flesh reap corruption," etc. (Gal. vi. 7, 8.)

CHAPTER II.

THE ENSLAVING POWER OF TOBACCO.

"If the Son therefore shall make you free, ye shall be free indeed."—John viii. 36.

"And the truth shall make you free."—John viii. 32.

But are tobacco smokers and chewers free ? Alas, there are but very few forms of bondage so galling as that of the tobacco consumer. How many of them often make the sad confession, "I would give up the habit if *I could.*" Is this Gospel freedom ? Is this liberty from enslaving habits ? Verily not. "An old man, who had borne an irreproachable character up to the age of seventy-two, was lately brought before one of the tribunals of Paris for steal-

ing a piece of lead worth eight cents. He admitted that
he was wholly without means, and for the first time in his
life knew not where to find a single sou ; but it was not
hunger that drove him to steal. After considerable ques·
tioning on the part of the judge as to what could be stronger
than hunger, he confessed it was *tobacco for his pipe.*
" Tobacco, monsieur judge !" said he, growing violent. " I
have the misery to be a hopeless smoker ! I smoke at
waking ; I smoke while eating ; I cannot sleep without
smoking till the pipe falls from my mouth. Tobacco costs
me six cents a day. When I have none I am frantic. I
cannot work, nor sleep, nor eat. I go from place to place
raging like a mad dog. The day I stole the lead, I had
been without tobacco twelve hours ! I searched the day
through for an acquaintance of whom I could beg a pipeful.
I could not, and resorted to crime as a less evil than I was
enduring. The need was stronger than I !"

So fearfully enslaving is the habit that its victims when
deprived of the weed for a while, will do almost anything
to get a quid, or pipeful of tobacco. A brute in human
form, named William Biddlescombe, was convicted by a
magistrate at Portsmouth, England, and sentenced to three
months' imprisonment for skinning a living small terrier
dog, and his only assigned reason for his cruelty was, that
he wanted the skin for a tobacco pouch ! ! !

" The Danes," writes the Brussels correspondent of the
Irish Times, " are passionately fond of smoking. The
punishment of death cannot be inflicted upon Danish
criminals unless they confess their crimes ; and the with·
holding of tobacco is said to frequently lead to an acknow-
ledgment of guilt, and, indeed, on some occasions to this
confession when the accused are *really innocent*, because
the beloved weed is no longer denied them. We have

heard," continues the writer, "of men dying for their country, for their creed, for their love, but it is strange to hear of martyrs to a deleterious plant."

Said a young man: "I believe my pipe does me harm; I feel it is injuring me; but were I certain that it would curtail my life by fifteen years, I could not give it up!!" How distressing to hear such a statement from a free-born son of Britain! "I am a slave to tobacco," says a lawyer, "and I will give a hundred dollars to be told how to get rid of it without killing me!" "I have resolved to be free a thousand times," says another, "but I am still a slave, a hopeless slave!" A deacon, on his death-bed, made the following painful statement: "I thank God, that as my last sickness has now come, I shall get rid of my hankering for tobacco!" The late Rev. George Trask writes: "I have known men to dream and rage about tobacco as madmen, when deprived of it. I have known men so enslaved that use it they would in parlors, in churches, in temperance meetings, in defiance of all remonstrance, in defiance of all decency. And one lodge of the Sons of Temperance (?) as I certainly know, passed a resolution that they would not lay aside their tobacco even during the hour they were convened for temperance purposes. I have known a temperance lecturer of great distinction positively refuse to lecture until he had been furnished with a pipe of tobacco to screw his nerves up to the point of eloquence. I know an excellent clergyman who assured me that he had sometimes wept like a child when putting a quid of tobacco in his mouth, under a sense of his degradation and bondage to this filthy habit. I saw a man who told me that tobacco was the dearest thing he had on earth—dearer than wife, child, church or state."

"I can name a clergyman who was much enslaved to his

snuff'; he sometimes reproved a neighbor who was a drunkard. At length the drunkard said to him, If you will give up your snuff, I will give up my rum. The bargain was made. But within forty-eight hours the clergyman was in perfect anguish for his snuff. He set a spy over the drunkard to watch for his downfall. When told that the fatal cup had passed his lips, he flew to his snuff-box with the fury of a maniac, made himself idiotic, and died a fool! Tell us which was the greater drunkard? Or, as sin is the point in debate, which was the greatest sinner? 'Dear sir,' we said to a brother clergyman, 'do, I pray you, give up tobacco.' 'Not I, not I,' was his reply, 'I will use it if it shortens my life seven years. I will smoke while I live.' If this is not slavery, what is slavery? Is it not a sin to practise a habit which makes an abject slave? An eminent minister once said, '*I would lay down one hundred pounds gladly at any time if I could give up smoking!.*' A woman in Essex county, a Christian professor, called for her snuff-box in her dying agonies, on the verge of eternity! Weeping friends witnessed her passion strong in death! Her last words were, "Nuff, nuff, give me nuff'!'"

There is many a man who would see widows and orphans, and even his *own* wife and children, suffer long for want of bread to eat, rather than leave off tobacco, if he had no other means, and devote the money for its purchase to their supply of bread.

This is a startling, and yet a tangible truth; and one which should look every tobacco slave in the face. Nine out of ten would sooner endure the sight of starvation in others than the teasings of this denied lust.

CHAPTER III.

THE IDOLATRY OF TOBACCO HABITS.

"Thou shalt have no other gods before me."—EXODUS xx. 3.

IT is computed that over three hundred millions worship this filthy idol ! ! "When many of the tobacco consumers get into trouble, or under any cross or affliction, instead of looking to God for support, the pipe or the twist is applied to with quadruple earnestness ; so that four times, I might say, in some cases, ten times, the usual quantity is consumed on such occasions. What a comfort is the weed in time of sorrow ! What a support in time of trouble ! In a word, what a god !"—*Dr. A. Clarke.*

Rev. George Trask, states the following : "For over thirty years, an old gentleman of St. Albans, Vt., has made a practice of getting out of bed every night at eleven, twelve, two, and four o'clock to *enjoy a comfortable smoke.* Few worship their God night and day. We are commanded to *pray* without ceasing, but this old tobacco user has misinterpreted the command, and *smokes* without ceasing. What a reproof to those who profess to worship the true God ! This poor soul, in order to finish his course with joy, sacrifices sleep. It is his meat and drink to obey the commands of his pipe. Another feature—he does it in succession, needs not a 'revival' to quicken his energies. He obeys one command, he has no other god but this ; he has no intercessor between him and his god, as they are on good terms. In all probability he will never forsake his god, or his god forsake him. He offers incense to this god night and day." Are there not thousands who are guilty of the same sin?

"That object for which we sacrifice most, we love most, and the object we love most is our god. Now, if this object be other than Jehovah, our service to it is idolatry. The confirmed tobacco slave does love stronger and sacrifice more for this weed than any other object in the universe. The man whose means are limited, who cannot afford luxuries for his family, cannot spare means for religious books, or his church paper, and not a cent to support Christ's cause, has plenty which he metes out with a lavish hand to gratify his craving appetite. This has become to him the prince of appetite, for he will gratify it before any other. He loves this sickening filth better than the choicest sweetmeats—sweeter to him than honey, and richer than the most luscious fruits."—*J. L. Benton*. Many a professor of religion, if worse came to worse, would drop his minister, his church, and even his Bible, with less ado than he would relinquish his pipe. God says: "Thou shalt have no other gods before me." But the common use of tobacco is idolatry—a violation of the above command, and hence it is a *sin*.

CHAPTER IV.

TOBACCO AND HARD TIMES.

"Give an account of thy stewardship."—LUKE xvi. 2.

THE consumption of this weed squanders over $1,000,000-000! America uses annually over one-half, or at least, $600,000,000! This would support all charitable institutions, and feed and clothe all the poor. The cost of one cigar per day, at 5 cts. would at 7 per cent., compound interest, amount in ten years to $252.16; in twenty years to $748.15; in thirty years to $1,034!!!

Tobacco clothes many poor men's children with rags, and does much to fill poor-houses. Tobacco and liquors cost enough to evangelize the world; they are the most fruitful sources of debt. Scripture plainly shows that we are only *stewards* of the things of this world; that therefore we are not to use and spend our money and property in any way or for anything that will not be acceptable unto God; in short, that we are not at liberty to waste a single cent, or squander the smallest item of our substance. If, therefore, we indulge in wasteful unnecessary expenditure, we use our means contrary to God's will and such an act becomes a sin —a *financial* sin. It would be accounted a wicked and wanton thing for a man to go and burn down his barns and dwelling house; in fact, such a deed would meet with severe retribution at the hands of the law. But the tobacco consumer spends his money—in many cases hard earned money—on tobacco, and then either sets fire to it, or chews it and throws it away! How frightfully large the sum of

money annually wasted by tobacco users is, let the following facts and figures show. The present annual production
of tobacco has been estimated by an English writer at
4,000,000,000 pounds. This is smoked, chewed, and
snuffed. Suppose it all made into cigars, one hundred to
the pound, it would produce 400,000,000,000. Four
hundred billions of cigars. Allowing this tobacco unmanu-
factured to cost on the average ten cents a pound, and we
have $400,000,000 expended every year in producing a
noxious deleterious weed. At least one and a half times as
much more is required to manufacture it into a marketable
form, and dispose of it to the consumer. If this be so, then
the human family expend *every year* one thousand millions
of dollars in the gratification of an acquired habit, or one
dollar for every man, woman and child upon the earth!
This sum would build two railroads around the earth, at a
cost of twenty thousands dollars per mile, or sixteen railroads from the Atlantic to the Pacific! It would build
one hundred thousand churches, costing $10,000 each; or
half a million of school-houses, costing $2,000 each; or one
million of dwellings, costing $1,000 each! It would
employ one million of preachers and one million of
teachers, giving each a salary of $500! It would support
three and one-third millions of young men at college, giving
each $300 per annum for expenses! At the late New
England Methodist Episcopal Conference held in Massachusetts, 1877, Bishop Harris is said to have expressed the
opinion that "the Methodist Church spends more for
chewing and smoking than it gives towards converting the
world." This is a sad statement to make of a large
religious body.

After fully forming the habit, a person will chew about
two inches of light plug per day. For convenience we will

say one foot a week, or fifty-two feet in a year, which will amount in fifty years to two thousand six hundred feet, or nearly *half a mile*. At present prices this is worth two cents per inch, which gives the neat little sum of six hundred and twenty-four dollars, which if deposited in the savings bank instead of the tobacconist's till, would have given the chewer a fine farm, instead of eighteen or twenty bushels of useless quids !

But suppose the man is a smoker, and indulges in cigars —very moderately, we will say only three per day, each four inches long, and costing two cents apiece. Each day he will consume a foot of tobacco, at an expense of six cents, or seven feet in a week, thirty per month, and three hundred and sixty-five feet a year—costing twenty-one dollars and ninety cents. In fifty years he will burn eighteen thousand two hundred and fifty feet, which would make a cigar three and a half miles long, costing one thousand and ninety-five dollars. Set upon end it would be higher than Mont Blanc.

Dr. Talmage says : "Put into my hand the moneys wasted in tobacco in Brooklyn, and I will support three orphan asylums as grand and beautiful as those already established. Put into my hand the money wasted in tobacco in the United States, and I will feed, clothe and shelter all the suffering poor on this continent. The American Church gives $5,500,000 a year for the evangelization of the heathen, and American Christians spend $600,000,000 in tobacco."

How can any man's complaint of *hard times* be entitled to the sympathy and beneficence of right-minded people while he is guilty of such wastefulness as this? Let such men cease from this sinful expenditure, and then their cry of poverty will be worthy of some consideration.

CHAPTER V.

TOBACCO INJURES THE MENTAL POWERS.

"Jesus said unto him, Thou shalt love the Lord thy God with all thy heart, and with all thy soul, and with all thy *mind*."— MATTHEW xx. 37.

IT is a recognized principle in nature *that whatever enfeebles the body must in the same degree enfeeble the mind.* "A sound mind in a sound body," is the physiological law. This *every tobacco user violates:* for it can be most conclusively shown, both by medical testimony and multiplying facts, that tobacco—by poisoning the blood and deranging the whole system—does, in thousands of instances, not only induce physical weakness and disease, but, sooner or later, extinguish life.

1. *Its general deleterious effects upon the mind.* It is a common notion among certain classes that the use of tobacco is a great help to the inventive and imaginative faculty. Let all those who hold this opinion read the following "Confessions of an Old Smoker":

"The effects of tobacco upon the brain are in some measure analogous to those produced by opium, only the mischief is of a milder form. It is not, however, the less real. At first there is a feeling of pleasurable excitement, which, *for a time*, does unquestionably aid the inventive and imaginative faculty. But the *ultimate* and the most *lasting* effects must be taken into account, and these my own experience has proved to be evil, and only evil. For the brain is rendered all the more feeble and apathetic *in its general state* by the *temporary* excitement produced by tobacco. I found a pipe or two very helpful for any great effort—very stimulating while the immediate effect of the weed was felt; but I was conscious that when *that* had passed away I was left with a brain less disposed to mental effort than ever. And it has become clear to me that, in *the whole of its influence,* the pipe is unfriendly to *general mental activity.* The man who smokes will do, *in the gross,* less intellectual work than a man of the same capacity will do who abstains from tobacco. I write positively on this view of the question, because experience has demonstrated the truth of what I affirm. It is a complete delusion to smoke with a view to increase the amount of brain work. How clearly is this proved by the simple fact that, without their pipe, confirmed smokers can do nothing! Set them to work, poor fellows, on some knotty and difficult question, and deny them their pipe, and their brain will refuse its office; their mental faculties will be as cloudy as the smoke in which they love to luxuriate, and they will soon lay down the pen in despair! They must have their pipes to *stimulate* the brain! They must smoke until the deadly and unnatural narcotic has done *its* work and then they can do *theirs!* This is no caricature, but a true picture. But what is the result (the whole result, I mean)? Why, that the brain is becoming more and more enfeebled, and its ordinary standard of activity diminished by every repetition of the temporarily exciting process. I was thunderstruck by observing how often the predictions of medical men were fulfilled in cases in which they had warned inveterate smokers of the mischiefs that would ensue from their devotion to this habit. I observed that many great smokers became prematurely old and infirm; that others were the victims of nervous petulence and irritability; that some became confirmed hypochondriacs; while many sank under that baneful malady, softening of the brain, and became idiots for the rest of their days! Tobacco has done all this in the case of several Christians and ministers of the Gospel. It has destroyed many a brain and many an intellect that has been devoted to the study and elucidation of eternal truth. It was the *false* idea that I should be able to get through more mental work in my lifetime, if I smoked, that lead me to devote myself to the practice; but it was a deep conviction, slowly and most unwillingly formed, that by smoking I was enfeebling my reason and sapping the energies of all my mental faculties, which eventually compelled me to abandon that habit."

"The pupils of the Polytechnic School in Paris have recently furnished some curious statistics bearing on tobacco. Dividing the young gentlemen of that college into two groups, the smokers and the non-smokers, it is shown that the smokers have proved themselves in the various competitive examinations far inferior to the others. Not only in the examinations on entering the school are the smokers in a lower rank, but in various ordeals they have to pass during the year, the average rank of the smokers had constantly fallen, and not inconsiderably; while the men who did not smoke enjoyed a cerebral atmosphere of the clearest kind."—*Dublin Medical Press.*

At other schools and colleges of France, the non-smokers have acquitted themselves at the examinations far better than those who used tobacco; they were healthier, closer students, and consequently better scholars. Smoking was therefore prohibited in all public seminaries in France.

Wm. Parker, M.D., of New York, says of tobacco: "It is ruinous in our schools and colleges, where it *dwarfs body and mind.*"

"I mention a curious fact," says Prof. Lizars, "which requires only to be tried to be proved;—that no smoker can think steadily, or continuously, on any subject while smoking. He cannot follow out a train of ideas;—to do so he must lay aside his pipe."

Dr. James Copland says: "Smoking tobacco weakens the nervous power, favors a dreamy, imaginative and imbecile state of mind, produces indolence and incapacity for manly or continuous exertion, and sinks its votary into a state of careless or maudlin inactivity, and selfish enjoyment of his vice."

Many observers on the Continent have noticed the inferior attainments of the students who smoke. Says Dr. Murray: "My own personal experience and observation among medical students is supported by the result of examinations for law and divinity, smokers having been found behind non-smokers in mental calibre."

"Within half a century no young man addicted to the use of tobacco has graduated at the head of his class in Harvard College, though five out of six of the students have used it. The chances, you see, were five in six that a smoker or chewer would graduate at the head of his class, if tobacco does not harm. But during half a century not one victim of tobacco was able to come out ahead. If a man wishes to train for a boat race, his trainer will not let him use tobacco, because it weakens his brain and muscles so that he cannot win. If a young man wishes to train for a long walk—say a hundred miles in twenty-four hours—his trainer will not let him touch a cigar, because he knows that the young chap will not be able to hold out in such a long walk. If a young fellow would prepare to play a fine game of billiards, while he is training for the tournament his trainer will not let him touch tobacco. And, as you see from the experience in Harvard College, if a man will train himself to graduate from a college with honor, he must not use tobacco. It is a powerful poison, and the brain cannot escape if it be used in any form."—*Dio Lewis, M.D.*, in "*Dr. Holbrook's Hygiene of the Brain and Nerves,*" *New York.*

The *Phrenological Journal* says : "Half the old tobacco users one meets are in a state of semi-imbecility. Their memory is leaky, moral sense blunted, general disposition impaired and tone of both body and mind let down."

2. *Loss of Memory.*—Loss of memory takes place in an extraordinary degree in the smoker, much more so than in the drunkard, evidently from tobacco acting more on the brain than alcohol. An eminent French savant had, for many years been a snuff-taker. He was conscious that the habit injured him. He quit repeatedly, but always began again. His daily allowance became larger and he noticed a rapid decay of the memory. "He had learned some 1,500 root words in each of several languages, but found them gradually dropping out of his mind, so as to necessitate frequent recurrence to dictionaries. At last he summoned resolution to break finally with the use of tobacco in any form, and after six years of abstinence writes as follows : 'It was for us the commencement of a veritable resurrection of health, mind and memory ; our ideas have become more lucid, our pen quicker, and we have seen gradually return that army of words which had run away. Our memory, in a word, has recovered all its riches, all its sensibility.' "

Dr. Rush states that the father of Massilac lost his memory at the age of forty-five, through the excessive use of snuff.

Dr. Cullen cites several instances in which tobacco induces loss of memory, fatuity, and other symptoms of a weakened or prematurely senile state of mind.

The Duke of Wellington, in his French campaign, complained of the excessive use of tobacco by his soldiers, and attempted to restrain it for the above reason.

In Dr. William Henderson's work on "Plain Rules for Improving Health," second edition, the following case is given: "One gentleman, from having been one of the most healthy and fearless men, became one of the most timid. He could not present a petition, much less say a word concerning it though he was a practising lawyer. He was afraid to be left alone at night." All through the use of tobacco!

"Melancholia (a species of insanity of which extreme melancholy, and nervous depression, is the characteristic) I have found resulting from excessive smoking. I have a case now under my care in which the patient first exhibited a want of memory, with extreme melancholy; then loss of reasoning power; next, inability to comprehend; and he now lives simply by instinct. Still, he sticks to his pipe!"—*Dr. Brewer.*

3. *Cowardice.*—Eminent physicians say that patients addicted to tobacco-smoking are in spirit cowardly, and deficient in manly fortitude to undergo any surgical operation, however trifling, proposed to relieve them from the suffering of other complaints.

It is well known that the Turks, in their recent wars, have not displayed as much courage as they did in the days of the Sultans Othman, Orchan, Amurath the First, and Bajazet. Hence many potentates, both in Europe and Asia, have forbidden their soldiers the use of tobacco "It is stated that the Sikhs, now named the Punjabees, never smoke tobacco, it being contrary to their religion. I may ask, are there any soldiers in India equal to the Sikhs? At Chillianwallah, at Moodkee, at Ferozshah, at Aliven, at Moelton, at Sobraon, no soldiers behaved better."

CHAPTER VI.

TOBACCO LEADS TO INSANITY.

"Thou shalt love the Lord thy God with all thy strength, and with all thy *mind*," etc.—MATT. xx. 37.

IT is a sad but incontrovertible fact that thousands of the human race become perfectly insane through the use of tobacco. We give a few facts in point. Says Dr. Wood-ward: "Tobacco produces insanity, I am fully confident."

Dr. Campbell, a medical superintendent of a lunatic asylum in New South Wales, says: "After exercising my profession for forty years, with no inconsiderable experience of the so-called diseases of the mind, I may be allowed to speak with some confidence on a habit which has consigned thousands to the mad-house, and hundreds of thousands to the rankling affliction of incurable diseases in the stomach and associated organs."

An eminent professor in one of the New England medical colleges, not many years ago, died in a mad-house, his madness being the consequence of snuffing.

An intoxicated soldier swallowed his saliva impregnated with tobacco, awoke in strong convulsions, and nearly became insane.

Miss Dix, the distinguished philanthropist, refers to eight cases of insanity produced by the use of tobacco in one asylum in Massachusetts.

Dr. Kirkbridge, in his report of Pennsylvania Hospital for the Insane, for 1849, states that "two cases in men and five in women were caused by the use of opium, and four in men by the use of tobacco."

Dr. Lizars gives the following case which shows that tobacco and not drink was the cause of insanity. A gentleman about thirty-five years of age, long addicted to drinking, smoking and chewing, became quite fatuous, and subject to fits closely resembling epilepsy. He was removed to a lunatic asylum, where the ardent spirits were first given up; but no change for the better for six months. The smoking tobacco was then reduced, when some little improvement took place ; and when both the smoking and chewing were reduced a great amendment followed, and when totally given up the fits ceased, and he became perfectly sane. He mentions five cases of insanity through tobacco.

Dr. Rubio, a French physician, calculates that in Europe the average consumption of tobacco is seventy ounces per head, per annum ! and he states that there is a frightful increase of insanity, proportioned to the increased consumption of tobacco. According to the researches of a high medical authority, recently, it is proved that one person out of every three hundred of the population of England and Wales, is either idiotic or insane. It appears also, that this frightful increase of idiocy and insanity lies chiefly among the young, and is ascribed in a great measure to the increase of tobacco smoking among boys.

The New York *Evening Post* says : "The case of M. O'C——, the Fair Haven groceryman who was taken to the almshouse a day or two ago, is a sad one. He is only twenty-eight years old, and has a wife and two children. He became an habitual and inveterate smoker, and his nervous system became so affected that his brain was injured, and insanity followed. Dr. Francis Bacon and other physicians warned him of his danger of smoking so much, but he failed to give up the habit. He was sent to the Middletown Asylum, and there deprived of the means of gratifying his appetite, improved, and was discharged as cured. But once out, he again resorted to narcotic stimulants, and again became insane. This is the second time he has been sent to the almshouse."

A very important fact, illustrative of the relation of tobacco and insanity, has recently been brought to light in France by a paper laid before the Academy of Science—namely, that insanity increases in proportion to the amount of tobacco used. Thus it is said between 1812 and 1832 (twenty years) the tax on tobacco produced twenty-eight millions of francs, and the lunatic asylum contained eight thousand patients. Since that time the tobacco revenue has reached the sum of one hundred and eighty millions of francs, and lunatics and paralytic patients have reached to forty-four thousand.

The New York *World*, in a late issue, asserts that in nine cases out of eleven, where insanity has resulted from inebriation, the primary cause was smoking. It also gives a list of patients in insane asylums, under treatment for confirmed inebriation, resulting in insanity, who preceded whiskey by tobacco smoking:

Bloomingdale Asylum.	out of 100			87
Flatbush	"	"	64	49
Trenton	"	"	56	48
Columbus	"	"	74	62

The *American Presbyterian* observes: "We have heard with great pain, of the death by suicide of Rev. John Howard, pastor of the Presbyterian church in Woodstock, Va. He was a man of deep piety, of uncommonly gentle spirit, and a member of a much respected family circle in Richmond. His theological studies were pursued at the Union Theological Seminary in New York, where his amiable spirit and gentlemanly demeanor attracted the affection of his fellow-students. Of a sensitive, nervous organization, and a hard student, it is supposed that the excessive use of tobacco aided to produce insanity."

The late Rev. George Trask gives the following sad cases : "He knew a brother minister of ripe talents and splendid oratory. He learned to smoke. His talents were dimmed and his admirers forsook him. He took the cup. The days of this eloquent young clergyman were ended in ignominy. A life which had promised to be happy and illustrious was brought to a miserable close. His intemperate habits killed his wife, it was supposed, and made a beggar of his child. *He died in a mad-house, blaspheming the very Saviour he had preached.*"

He mentions another, Rev. John S——, pastor of a New England church, who persisted in the use of tobacco, till delirium set in and he said he must have more or die. After seven years of suffering, "he became an imbecile and died a fool!" "Mr. G——, a parishioner, was soon after buried. He had promised to give up rum if his pastor gave up tobacco. For a while each tried to abstain, but the habit which was first a hair, was found to have become a cable. One died a drunkard, and the other a tobacco suicide."

"In one asylum we found that every patient save one was a tobacco user previous to coming there. In another, we found three insane clergymen, rendered so, we were told by the superintendent, by the baneful power of tobacco. Painful spectacle ! As we entered their room they clamored for tobacco. They reiterated their cry, 'Tobacco ! tobacco !'"

A certain eminent clergyman had to be shut up in an insane asylum for twenty years, through the use of tobacco. Another died insane from the same cause.

Prof. Thwing records the case of a minister who went raving mad through the use of the cursed weed. He was shut up in a lunatic asylum for many years. He there breathed a fetid atmosphere, paced the floor of confined halls, stared upon the outside world through iron grates, cursed himself, cursed his wife and children, and in his wild ravings "dealt damnation round the land," thus day and night champing tobacco as a fretted horse champs his bit. He once was pacing his room as he had aforetime year after year, when a change came over him. He stopped abruptly, and in a sort of soliloquy exclaimed, "Why am I here? What brought me here? What binds me here?" His soul bursting with indignation, he cried aloud, "Tobacco! tobacco!" He walked backward and forward; then, bursting into tears, he cast the last foul plug through the iron grates, and looking upward to God he said, "O God, help! help! I will use no more." He was cured by giving up the weed.

Uncle Toby relates the case of a youth whom he went to visit in New England—a lunatic through the use of tobacco:

"All on a sudden James Dixey, the young maniac, was in motion; he rattled down the staircase, and whirled around the room with the fury of a tornado.

"His eyes were distended, wild, and flashing fire. His skin was greasy, and the hue of dirty brass, or a boiled chicken; his muscles were distorted, his hair clotted, and his attitude, expression, and all, was obscene, and awfully loathsome.

"The tobacco demon—I believe tobacco hath a devil, and the devil hath it—I say the tobacco demon who had possession of this mad boy was by no means bashful or retiring; he cried out, 'Tobacco! tobacco!' with an unearthly scream, that seemed to well-nigh raise the roof,

"Tobacco he would have at any rate. When not furnished by his parents he would beg it from door to door. When he could not beg it he would steal it. When he could not get it in one town he would go to another, and there was no peace, day or night, beneath the roof when the young maniac was out of tobacco!"

There are about 70,000 lunatics in America. More than 15,000 of these were made insane by the use of tobacco!

CHAPTER VII.

TOBACCO AND DISEASE.

"Thou shalt not kill."—Exodus xxv. 13.

If tobacco is useful or necessary to health. we need not be scrupulous as to the amount we spend upon it. If it were simply for the gratification of an animal appetite, without adding to, or detracting from the sum of our health or happiness, to lay out expense on such an article would seem to us all at best a childish folly. But if it can be shown to be positively hurtful, prejudicial to the vital functions, endangering health and shortening life, then to expend money on it is worse than folly—it is madness, and should be classed with what is expended on the cups of the drunkard—an expense to which he is impelled by a depraved appetite, while he knows it is hurrying himself to ruin, and preparing himself for beggary.

Dr. Trask, the apostle of the anti-tobacco reform, says: "I can specify on sound medical authority more than fifty diseases that spring from this vile narcotic, or which are greatly intensified by its use."

Dr. Moiselli, of Turin, gives elaborate statistics to prove that since 1827 suicides have increased in all civilized countries from 48 to 150 per each million of inhabitants; and this increase is much in accordance with the increase in the use of tobacco.

Dr. Cole testifies : "Tobacco is more deadly to life than alcohol ; the latter is doing a greater evil to the innocent portion of the public, but the former is more deadly on its own victims, while the fire of alcohol burns with a mighty blaze. Tobacco burns long and deep in the fountain of life ; the one soon exhausts itself : the other stealthily eats away the cords of life by imperceptible degrees of its victim, until in time he dies in his sleep or falls dead in the street."

To give an elaborate description of all the manifold injuries the use of tobacco does to health, would be impossible in a chapter of this length, but we append the following which is the result of a long and careful investigation of medical statements on the subject in question :

1. *Dizziness of the head*, caused by irregular supply of arterial blood in the brain, is a common result of the free use of tobacco.

Says Dr. Mussey : " A friend of mine in this town, who has made a constant use of tobacco by chewing for more than thirty years of his life, was prevailed upon a few months ago to lay it aside, in consequence of having constant vertigo (dizziness) ; he is now well, and all who knew him are astonished to witness the increase of his flesh since he desisted from its use."

2. *Debility and Nausea.*—In whatever form it may be taken, a portion of the active principles of tobacco, mixed

3

with the saliva, invariably finds its way into the stomach, and disturbs or impairs the functions of that organ. As long as men persist in the habit, they must expect to experience, and that not seldom, that relaxation and weakening in the stomach, and that desire to vomit, which is so peculiar to sea-sickness, or whenever poison of a virulent strong kind has been taken.

"The pain which the weed at first inflicts is Jehovah's warning voice, saying, 'Taste not, touch not, handle not!' And can a Christian man, or any man, in fact, refuse to hear that warning voice without sin? I answer most respectfully, and yet most firmly, No! There is no denying the fact, that this is nearly the experience of every smoker, no matter at what period of life he may begin. But ought not this one fact to settle the question, whether the use of tobacco be lawful or not?"—*From "Confessions of an Old Smoker."*

William Parker, M.D., also says: "I do not place my individual self in opposition to tobacco, but science in the form of physiology and hygiene, is opposed to it, and science is the expression of God's will in the government of His work in the universe. Do you say, 'It never made me sick—I loved it from the first?' Then you exhibit the dreadful fact, that this accursed appetite may be entailed by the parent upon the child."

3. *Indigestion.*—Eminent medical men unite in testifying that the use of tobacco is one of the chief causes of this fearful disease.

Dr. Prout observes: "The severe and peculiar dyspeptic symptoms sometimes produced by inveterate snuff-taking are well known, and I have more than once seen such cases terminate fatally with malignant disease of the stomach and liver."

" Tobacco impairs the natural taste and relish for food, lessens the appetite, and weakens the power of the stomach."—*Dr. J. C. Warren.*

"It is a mistake to suppose that smoking aids digestion. The very uneasiness which it were desirable to remove, is occasioned either by tobacco itself, or by some other similar means. If tobacco facilitates digestion, how comes it that after laying aside the habitual use of it, most individuals experience an increase of appetite and of digestive energy, and an accumulation of flesh ?"—*Dr. Mussey.*

What an awful quantity of saliva is ejected through the mouth by tobacco users ! And how great is the injury they must do to themselves by the continued draining from their mouths of that necessary fluid a wise Creator has provided in their system !

Every medical man knows well that the saliva which is so copiously drained off by the infamous quid and the scandal-ous pipe, is the first and greatest agent which nature employs in digesting the food.

After a chewer has become rooted and grounded in his habit he will spit, on an average, twice in five minutes, and half a teaspoonful at a time, making 24 expector-ations in an hour, or about 240 in a day, which will amount to 120 drachms, or about a pint. This will give 360 pints, or 45 gallons in a year. Almost one and a half barrels ! If his vitality stands this drain for fifty years, he will have lost 2,250 gallons, or over 71 barrels—enough to fill a good-sized cistern. Estimating a pint as weighing a pound he will lose seven pounds per week, or 365 pounds per year, and 18,250 pounds, or over nine tons in fifty years ! Can we wonder that the tobacco user is thin and haggard-looking, when he spits away his own weight in less than six months ?

"It is a delusion under which some smokers labor, that their peculiar and beloved habit aids digestion. They say that, 'If their bowels are obstinately sluggish, an extra pipe or two will generally give them relief.' This I know from experience to be true, but I also know from experience that it is not the whole truth; for the following additional facts must be remembered. The very sluggishness of the bowels, of which smokers are so apt to complain, is produced by smoking; just as the habitual use of purgatives will be sure to cause indigestion. Again, the relief secured by taking 'an extra pipe or two,' is only temporary, while the entire and permanent result is an aggravation of the derangement complained of, just as cathartics of extra strength only feed the malady which for a few days they alleviate. Of course, the stomach and bowels require a little time in order to recover their proper sensibility, which tobacco has for years been destroying. But let nature have time and fair play, and she will come right again, unless the mischief has become so serious as to assume an organic form; and then the sufferer will be better without tobacco. That smoking cannot aid digestion is self-evident. Its ultimate effect is to destroy the healthy sensibility of the coats of the stomach and bowels. And that such a process as this must be eventually ruinous to the health, who can doubt."—*From "Confessions of an Old Smoker."*

Sir B. Brodie says: "But the ill effects of tobacco are not confined to the nervous system. In many instances there is a loss of healthy appetite for food, the imperfect state of the digestion being soon rendered manifest by the loss of flesh and the sallow countenance."

4. *Amaurosis.*—Amaurosis is a disease of the eye, or of the nerve of vision. It is a serious disorder, difficult of cure

and often ending in permanent blindness. Of late the attention of medical observers has been directed to it as a common effect of tobacco.—*Gibbons' Tract.*

Mr. Jonathan Hutchinson has narrated several cases of amaurosis, the histories of which go far to establish the fact, that in each case the blindness was brought on by that rapidly increasing and, as it appears, baneful habit ; and in the *Medical Times and Gazette*, September 4th, the same distinguished surgeon has described another striking case of tobacco amaurosis, ending in absolute blindness, induced by eighteen months. The patient, aged fifty, a railway clerk, enjoyed good sight until January, 1867, and excellent general health, with the exception of a single attack of gout. He is a remarkably intelligent man ; was in former life a great reader, and says Mr. Hutchinson, " he tells me that since his affliction, he has been made acquainted with the particulars of many similar cases. I wish to ask especial attention to the fact that the man was smoking heavily, whilst taking no kind of alcoholic stimulants."

On this subject Dr. Drysdale remarks as follows : " The influence of tobacco on the eyesight is not well known. One of the symptoms produced in acute poisoning by tobacco is blindness ; and chronic poisoning gives rise to similar symptoms. Mackenzie, of Glasgow, first noticed that male patients affected with one species of amaurosis were mostly great lovers of tobacco. Hutchinson narrated, before the Royal Medical and Chirurgical Society of London, thirty-seven cases of a species of amaurosis, where twenty-three of the patients were great smokers ; and Woodsworth has confirmed these views of Mackenzie and Hutchinson. " In one week I saw (in 1874) at the Royal London Ophthalmic Hospital, two cases of tobacco amaurosis in young men, neither of whom had attained the age of thirty. The first had chewed continually ; and the second had smoked the enormous quantity of one ounce of shag tobacco daily. Both were completely and irretrievably blind from this dangerous habit." But weak sight is also commonly caused by snuffing as well as by smoking and chewing. Tobacco amaurosis is now much more common than it used to be. Mr. Couper, of the Royal London Ophthalmic Hospital, says that patients with tobacco amaurosis describe themselves as always living in a dim light, even at noon-day. Mr. George Critchett, the great London authority of diseases on the eye, states that he is constantly consulted by gentlemen for commencing blindness caused solely by smoking. which he condemns, therefore, in unqualified terms, as most dangerous to human health. Dr. Richardson confirms these statements and mentions, as the effect of tobacco, " dilatations of the pupils of the eye, confusion of vision, bright lines, luminous or cobweb specks, and long retention of images on the retina."

" My observation of eye diseases, extending through a period of more than twenty-five years, has convinced me that, besides the pernicious effects of tobacco in other respects (which we shall not now enumerate), greatly impaired vision, not unfrequently blindness, has been occasioned in the use of this agent, denominated in the books a narcotic poison. My experience in this regard is corroborated by that of those who have enjoyed the largest opportunities for investigating this subject."—*William Dickinson, M.D.*, in the *Central Christian Advocate.*

J. W., a coach-builder, upwards of fifty years of age, had smoked for thirty years, generally two ounces of tobacco a week, when he became so blind as to be unable to work, or even walk through a crowded street. He applied to an eye dispensary where the medical man who is considered a good oculist, told him that he labored under amaurosis, and prescribed accordingly.   After following his treatment for some time, and finding himself no better, he visited a neighboring city and consulted another oculist, who instantly detected tobacco to be the cause of his blindness, as if the obnoxious stench of the weed had led him at once to this conclusion.   J. W. instantly threw away tobacco forever, visited a relative in the Highlands where in a short time his vision returned, became clear, and enabled him to return to his business quite cured. A skilful English physician states that out of thirty-seven patients suffering from loss of sight by paralysis of the optic nerve, twenty-three were inveterate smokers.

Inflamed eyes, spasms of the eyelids, and cataract, are also caused by snuffing and sometimes by chewing.   "I may mention," says a correspondent, "that while travelling last month on a Danish steamer, I had much conversation on various subjects with a Belgian medical man, who informed me that he was then engaged, at the request of the Belgian Government, on a journey of observation and enquiry as to the causes of color blindness, an ocular affection, which, he said, is occasioning increasing anxiety, not merely in his own country, but especially in Germany, from its influence upon railway and other accidents, and also, to some extent, upon military inefficiency.   I asked the question—'What, so far as your investigations have proceeded, appears to be the main cause of this color blindness?'   He replied: 'The too general and excessive use of tobacco.'"

Says Dr. Griscomb: "The opinion has long been entertained that tobacco has been a frequent cause of loss of sight.   The diseased condition of the eyes produced by it is a species of amaurosis (paralysis of the optic nerve), commencing with symptoms of functional brain disease, and alterations of the supply of blood to the optic nerve and retina. These affections occur in large excess in adult males, being very infrequent to women, and a large portion of those who suffer from it, have been smokers."

Dr. Drysdale, senior physician to the Metropolitan Free Hospital, London, England, says: "I have seen several well-marked cases of nicotic blindness in young men under thirty who have chewed: for chewing is, of course, as it affords nicotine to the blood, much more rapidly poisonous than smoking; but the long continued smoking of shag tobacco, or, above all, of Cavendish tobacco, in quantities from half an ounce to an ounce daily, very frequently causes blindness in men at forty."

5. *Neuralgia.*—Strange as it may seem to some, the use of tobacco has frequently brought on this distressing pain. Dr. E. Johnson, of England, mentions an inveterate case of neuralgia in the heel, caused by chewing. Dr. Wood, of Philadelphia, mentions tobacco amongst the causes of this disease. It has also been traced in the head through the use of the weed, and other parts of the body have thus been affected. The late Chief Justice Richardson, of New Hampshire, says that he was once troubled with severe attacks of neuralgia, which confined him to his room for weeks with the most excruciating pains in his right side and breast. On his abandonment of the use of tobacco, this complaint entirely left him.

6. *It is Hurtful to the Teeth.*—"The common belief," says Dr. Warren, "that tobacco is beneficial to the teeth is, I apprehend, entirely erroneous. On the contrary, by poisoning and relaxing the vessels of the gums, it may impair the healthy condition of the vessel belonging to the

membranes of the socket, with the condition of which the
state of the tooth is closely connected." Tobacco arrests
toothache in some instances by its narcotic or killing power.
But anything that is capable of causing caries of the teeth
—which tobacco does—is liable also to induce toothache.
Tobacco softens the enamel of the teeth to such a degree
that they become worn off to the gums in numerous
instances. The young smoker may smile at the mention
of such an injury as this, but let him remember that the
teeth are too precious a means of preserving the body in
health to be ruthlessly sacrificed. That the smoking of
tobacco blackens and ultimately destroys the teeth of its
devotees, thousands of living witnesses can testify from sad
experience.

Says an old converted smoker: "I have known thoroughly hard smokers who, at forty years of age, have scarcely
had a sound tooth left in their heads. But this generally
brings with it other ailments. Imperfect mastication is
sure to produce indigestion; hence, you commonly find
that those who have destroyed their teeth by smoking are
terribly dyspeptic. Frequently, too, you find them martyrs
to toothache, tic douloureux or neuralgia. Let no one who
wishes to escape dyspepsia and its horrors throw away his
teeth by the use of tobacco."

The late Rev. G. Trask writes: "Tobacco acts disastrously on the gums. Its poisonous touch deadens the vitality
and causes the flesh to recede from the roots, leaving them
bare. It often acts disastrously on the enamel of the teeth
by perforating and blackening it: and the victim, instead
of presenting two rows of handsome grinders, presents you
with a mouth which reminds you of a sepulchre full of
dead men's bones."

"The idea that an acrid, biting, smutching poison, like

tobacco, preserves the teeth would be ridiculous were it
not pitiable.   It may be admitted that the poison, placed
on the thread-like throbbing nerve, may soothe it—in other
words make it drunk ; but to accomplish this the whole
magnificent network of nerve, from crown to toe, must, in
the nature of the case, be rendered more or less boozy or
stupid.   Which is worse, the remedy or the disease ?"

Says Dr. Mussey : " The opinion that the use of tobacco
preserves the teeth, is supported neither by physiology nor
observation."

" I have treated over one hundred cases of cancer this
year (1880), and out of that number were eighteen tobacco
cancers in the mouth.   Three out of the eighteen were
cured, and fifteen died.   One man had his tongue cut off."
—*Dr. A. L. W. Bowers.*

Dr. Warren, of Boston, agrees with Dr. Stone in his
opinion, and also affirms that " excessive smoking produces
cancerous affections of the tongue and lips."

Dr. Rush mentions a man in Philadelphia who lost all
his teeth by smoking.

The following is a testimony from a clergyman a hundred
years old and more : " In early life I commenced the practice of chewing tobacco, because I was told that it would
preserve my teeth, and prevent their aching.   The aching
was prevented ; but it early destroyed as fine a set of teeth
as was ever set in a man's head."

A friend observes : " One night I was crossing some
fields on my way home, and was suddenly seized with
the toothache.   I took some tobacco and put it into my
mouth, hoping to get rid of the pain ; but I had not gone
far before I felt giddy, and when I got within a short
distance of a stile, I fancied I could lay my hand on it, but
I reeled about and pitched headlong.   I repeated my efforts,

but the fact was, that I was a long way off the stile, although I thought myself near. Instead of reaching home at ten o'clock, I didn't get there till twelve. At the door I held the knob with one hand and rang the bell with the other. My wife tried to open the door, but as fast as she tried to open it, I pulled it back. At length she said, 'What do you mean by making such a fool of yourself at this time of night?' 'I can't help it; I am drunk, and can't stand upright. I've had the toothache, and, as I had no pipe with me, I chewed some tobacco, and I am completely drunk.' It was a long time," he adds, "before I could walk upstairs. But I took good care never to chew again for toothache." Gumboils and wasting of the gums are frequently the effects of using tobacco.

7. *Deafness and Earache.*—"Smoking and snuff-taking have a particularly noticeable effect on the hearing, and it may be noticed as a rule that old snuff-takers are more or less hard of hearing."

M. Triquet states that, in smokers and drinkers, an insidious and obstinate form of otitis (inflammation of the ear) frequently becomes developed. Dr. Mussey mentions the case of Mr. Cummings, in Plymouth, N.H., who, though he enjoyed at the age of twenty the best of health, commenced the use of snuff, and afterward, at the age of twenty-five, resorted to chewing and smoking. In this way he went on, for thirty years till he was nearly destroyed. The effects on his senses were striking. At the age of fifty-five he could not read a word in any book without spectacles; and he had already been in the use of them for several years. He had also been subject to a ringing and deafness in both ears for ten years, and at times the right ear was entirely deaf. "In about a month after quitting his snuff (which was the last thing he gave up), his hearing became correct, and none of his troubles with this organ ever returne l. It was many months, however, before he could dispense with spectacles ; but finally he got rid of them. At sixty-three his senses were keener, especially his eyesight, than those of most men at his age."

Dr. L. B. Coles says : "While travelling on the upper Mississippi, two cases of this kind came under my observation. They were both young men, between, probably, the ages of thirty and thirty-five. They had been hard smokers from early life. One was on his way for medical advice. On riding with him and investigating the history and nature of his case, it became my conviction that the seat of the trouble was in the auditory nerve, which had lost its electric energy ; and that it was the tobacco that had paralyzed its tone. It was here that its destructive agency had principally located itself. In the other case its direct attack on the nerves of hearing had demonstrated itself. The man stated that a few months since he suspended the use of tobacco for only a single month, and found his hearing essentially improved. But such was the strength of appetite, and his unwillingness to attribute the difficulty to the idol of his mouth, he entered upon its use again, and his hearing became as bad as before."

8. *Impaired Voice.*—"Tobacco when used in the form of snuff," says Dr. Rush, "seldom fails of impairing the voice by obstructing the air." Says another : " It is not the snuff-taker alone who injures his voice by tobacco. Smoking and chewing produce similar effects The smoke of tobacco contains many fine particles, which lodge in the passages. Who does not know how soon smoke of any kind, especially tobacco smoke, will darken or blacken a white surface ? Yet, how could it darken it except by depositing its fine dust upon it ? And is the membrane of

the nasal passages less likely to receive the filthy, poisonous deposit than any other surface? Do we wonder, then, why the voice should be affected, when the hollow nasal cavities are converted into so many sooty flues of a sooty chimney?" Dr. Allen, of Maine, says: "That tobacco is injurious to the voice, anyone can testify who has heard the harsh, thick, husky, mumbling, stammering, insonorous voice of the tobacco chewer." Who has not noticed the peculiar nasal twang among great users of snuff and tobacco? "One frequent cause of permanent loss of voice in modern times by public speakers, especially clergymen, is owing to the use of tobacco in some of its forms.'—*Dr. Woodward.*

Mr. J. H—— began to chew tobacco at an early age and used it freely. When about fifty-five years old he lost his voice, and was unable to speak above a whisper for three years. During the four or five years which preceded the loss of his voice, he used a quarter of a pound of tobacco in a week. He was subject to fits of extreme melancholy; for whole days he would not speak to any one, was exceedingly dyspeptic, and was subject to nightmare. Upon abandoning his tobacco his voice gradually returned, and was greatly benefited in many other respects.

9. *Epilepsy.*—This is another effect of the use of tobacco. A son of Mr. F , at the age of fifteen, was taken home from one of the public schools on account of having had several attacks of epilepsy. After a few months it was discovered during one of his attacks, that he had tobacco in his mouth. Directions were given for regulating his diet, and he was advised to omit the use of tobacco. While he abstained from the use of it he was free from any epileptic attack. The attack, however, frequently

returned, and on every occasion of the kind, tobacco was either found in his mouth or his pocket. The administration of medicine was finally given up as unavailing, and after dragging out ten years of a life useless to his friends and to himself, he died.

Another similar case occurred at Troy, N.Y., with this exception: The victim, after having been struck with epilepsy through the use of tobacco, became an idiot and died. Dr. Mussey, one of the most eminent surgeons of our country, has known this sad disease to result from the use of tobacco.

10. *Palsy or Paralysis.*—That thousands of tobacco users have brought on a very serious state of nervousness and paralysis by the use of the weed, themselves with others will frankly admit. How many of them we see scarcely able to put the pipe into their mouth without trembling like a leaf. That shaking of the hands shows too plainly what the much loved narcotic has done for them.

"It is painful to reflect on the numerous cases of apoplexy and paralysis which are occurring in the present day. We do not find these complaints simply attacking aged persons; neither youth or early manhood escapes. There is no more likely remote cause of these deplorable nervous maladies than tobacco smoking."—*Dr. Brewer.*

M. Jolly, inquiring into the general paralysis in France, discovered that it was the result of smoking. Dr. Martin, of Warrington, says: "Such cases were unknown in this country forty years ago. At that time there was much less smoking and much more drinking than in subsequent years."

"An intimate smoking friend of my own so suffered from shaking palsy of the hands, that the offer of £10,000 to fill his wineglass without spilling any would merely have caused his head to shake badly. To attempt shaving him would have been suicide. A few months ceasing to smoke the poison entirely cured his palsy."—*Dr. MacKenzie.*

A distinguished medical student at Brighton, England, has given a list of sixteen cases of paralysis produced by smoking, which came to his own knowledge in six months.

Dr. Brewer says: "I was once called upon to attend a young gentleman of good family who was suffering in this way; he had also lost all control over the lower half of his body, and was in a most pitiable condition. He had always lived an idle life, and been a great smoker from boyhood.

"I have another patient, a man sixty-eight years old, who has been suffering from shaking palsy for upward of two years. He cannot keep either of his limbs steady for a minute at a time, nor even his head. He has smoked tobacco for about fifty years.

"Not long ago, an admiral, whose nephew's legs were paralyzed, took him to a physician for consultation. While in the waiting-room, he perused a copy of the *Anti-Tobacco Journal* in which the *modus operandi* of tobacco in producing paralysis was explained, and on entering the consulting-room he said, 'I have brought my nephew, whose legs are paralyzed, to see if you can do anything for him; but from observations which I have been reading in the *Anti-Tobacco Journal*, I think smoking has caused paralysis.' 'Let me see him,' said the doctor; and he instantly confirmed the admiral's opinion."

Dr. Ledward, of Manchester, once told an audience at the end of an anti-tobacco lecture in that city, that he once had several patients, strong looking men, that no medicine would do any good unless they left off smoking, which they did, and all of them recovered their lost muscular power.

"Tobacco," says Dr. Levey, "enervates the intellect, plunges it into vagueness, and the free flow of ideas seems slackened. It is this nervous depression which gives to tobacco the epithet of soother and consoler." "It more or less affects body and mind," writes another, "and its victim becomes an eminently uneven creature—often in the condition of a steam engine, moving at the rate of fifty or a hundred miles an hour ; anon like the same engine, with a collapsed boiler, smashed up by the wayside."

According to Mr. Moreau, not a single case of general paralysis is seen in Asia Minor, where there is no abuse of alcoholic liquors, and where they smoke a kind of tobacco which is almost free from nicotine, or the peculiar poison in tobacco.

Dr. Shaw gives a case of paralysis agitans (shaking palsy), that beyond all doubt was caused by immoderate and long continued use of the weed. The patient was an elderly gentleman, who, for many years of life, could scarcely convey food to his mouth, although he was naturally, and by inheritance, one of the strongest and healthiest of men. He was finally carried off by a severe rheumatic attack. We have heard of three cases of palsy caused directly by the use of tobacco. "It is my business to point out to you all the various and insidious causes of general paralysis, and smoking is one of them. I know of no single vice that does so much harm as smoking. It is a snare and a delusion. It soothes the excited, nervous system at the time, to render it more irritable and more feeble ultimately."—Dr. Solly.

The following account of a paralytic in New York, was some time ago communicated by a gentleman to a public journal : "For thirty years he had been a daily smoker of the choicest cigars, but in all his other habits temperate and regular, and of excellent constitution—one who, of all men, would have laughed at the idea of tobacco killing him. Suddenly he was stricken with the progressive paralysis, characteristic of nicotine, and in one week he died. His death was pitiable. First sight was lost, then speech, then motion of the neck, then motion of the arms, and so on throughout the body, and he lay for a week unable to move or to make a sign, save a pitiful, tongue-less, inarticulate sound, which sometimes rose to almost frantic effort, all in vain to make known what he wished to say to his friends; for his consciousness and mental faculties were left unimpaired until two hours of the last, to aggravate to the utmost the horror of his situation—a living soul in a dead body. The sense of hearing was left unimpaired, so that he was conscious of all around him, while as incapable of communication with them as if dead, save by a slight sign of assent, or dissent, to a question. The doctors were fully agreed that tobacco was the sole cause of the stroke."

11. *Heart Disease.*—One of the most dreadful and yet common effects of tobacco using is partial paralysis of the nerves distributed to the heart; from this proceeds hurried and enfeebled action of that organ. This induces palpitations, and is frequently a chief cause of organic derangements, ending in fatal heart disease.

Monsieur Decaisne, in a communication to the French Academy of Science, states that in the course of three years, he met among 88 inveterate smokers, 21 cases of marked intermission of the pulse, occurring in men from 27 to 42 years of age, which could not be explained by any organic disease of the heart, thus proving it to be caused by a disturbance of the nerves controlling that organ. In

4

nine of these cases, when the use of tobacco was abandoned, the normal action of the heart was restored.

Dr. Marshall Hall mentions a case in the *Edinburgh Medical Journal* which almost terminated fatally; it was that of a young man, who, for his first essay, smoked two pipes.

Dr. Stone, of Troy, says it is the true cause of a large number of fatal cases of heart disease.

A physician once said, " We are accused of killing our patients by calomel. A thousand are killed by tobacco where one is killed by calomel."

Dr. Twitchell found that nearly all the cases of death during sleep, which came under his observation, were of men who had indulged largely in tobacco, and the correctness of his statements was confirmed by investigations made by the Boston Society for medical observation.

Dr. J. H. Kellog says : "The poison contained in a single pound of tobacco is sufficient to kill three hundred men, if taken in such a way as to secure its full effect. A single cigar contains poison enough to extinguish two human lives if taken at once."

The average life of operatives in tobacco factories is computed at four years. Dr. Kostral, physician to the Royal Tobacco factory in Moravia, reports that " of one hundred boys entering the works there, seventy-two fell sick during the first six months, while deaths frequently occur from the nicotine poisoning by inhaling the dust."

President Grant's lamentable death is attributed to the free use of cigars. Frederick III., late Emperor of Germany, is believed to have died from the effects of the same poison.

Dr. Jackson informs us of a minister who, after having used tobacco for many years, killed himself with the deadly poison. A post mortem examination was held. No evidence of diseased structure was exhibited in any of the internal organs except the heart. When the operators reached the heart and took it out, they found it nearly disorganized. The tenacious coherence of its fibres had entirely disappeared ; and one of the physicians present at the examination, wrote me that it could be picked to pieces with as much ease as a piece of fried liver.

12. *Delirium Tremens.*—This is one of the most fearful diseases with which sin avenges itself upon the human race. Dr. A. B. Spoor, of New York, a learned physician, says, that he is prepared to show that the horrible disease delirium tremens, has been ascribed to a wrong source—alcohol instead of tobacco. He says prior to the use of tobacco, delirium tremens was unheard of and unknown.

Dr. Lizars records three cases of this disease produced by tobacco alone. Drs. Mussey and Williams report similar cases. The lamented Geo. Trask says : " In the Marshall Infirmary in Troy, I saw a patient who could not rise from his seat without help ; when he was raised, however, he would stand by the hour trembling. On inquiry, he informed me that he had been in the habit of using two papers of tobacco daily, one of smoking and one of chewing."

Dr. Whitfield, of St. Thomas' Hospital, has seen three cases of delirium tremens induced by tobacco smoke alone.

A man died with this terrible disease in Monee, Ill., a few years ago, who was never known to use any kind of liquor, but was an inveterate user of tobacco."

Squire McGill, of Covington, Ky., died some time ago of delirium tremens, from the excessive use of tobacco and coffee.

A friend gives us a very striking case that came under his own notice, that was cured by giving up tobacco.

Says Dr. Mussey: "I was acquainted with a gentleman in Vermont who conscientiously abstained from all intoxicating drinks, yet died of delirium tremens from the excessive use of tobacco." Many similar cases might be given did space permit.

13. *Apoplexy.*—This disease is also a common effect of the deadly narcotic. In the *Dictionnarie des Sciences Medicales,* for 1821, two brothers are said to have smoked until they died of apoplexy—the one after smoking seventeen pipes, the other eighteen pipes. Dr. Lizars' book reports a sad case of apoplexy resulting from the use of tobacco. Dr. Cheyne, in speaking of snuffling, says: "I am convinced apoplexy is one of the evils of that disgusting practice." Dr. Hosac attributes the alarming frequency of apoplexy to the use of tobacco. Dr. Clay, of Manchester, England, says almost all whom he had known of late die of this dreadful disease, were inveterate snufflers. United States Secretary of the Navy Thompson, while at breakfast some time ago, was suddenly taken with a fainting fit, which lasted for some minutes. It was said he was stricken with apoplexy and paralysis. His physician thinks that his illness was caused by the excessive use of tobacco. In 1856, a committee from the Queen's College of Physicians, in London, in a report on the cause of death by apoplexy within the city, stated that the bills of mortality from this disease were very large, and that seven in nine cases of paralysis and apoplexy were caused by the use of tobacco. Of this number more than one-half was caused by snuffling. In confirmation of this, is the rarity with which this form of disease is met with in females.

Dr. Salmon says: "More people have died of apoplexy since the use of snuff, in one year, than have died of that disease in one hundred years before." Young people are taken off with apoplexy now, in contradistinction to the fact that old people used to be the only victims of this disease. This fact is proved by the Registrar-General's reports.

14. *Bronchitis.*—A somewhat peculiar form of this disease, known by a short, dry, hacking cough, is apt to be experienced by smokers.

15. *Cancer of the lower lip and tongue.*—This is a very general effect of tobacco. In his work on Tobacco, Dr. Lizars gives six cases of ulceration of the tongue, two of which ended fatally. In one case the victim suffered excruciating pain for several months. His tongue literally mouldered away. He could take no nourishment, his mouth and lower jaw being in a horrid state of ulceration. The doctor declares that "all the death-bed scenes and death-bed sufferings his medical adviser had ever witnessed were comparatively easy to the individual agonies and gaspings for breath of this kind and amiable man." The same book also mentions two cases of cancer of the tongue from the same cause, and says: "How many narrow escapes of having cancer of the tongue must every smoker have had, when we consider that everyone with a disordered stomach has had one or more pimples on his tongue, which, had they been irritated with pungent tobacco smoke, would in all probability have ended in ulceration, became cancerous, and ended fatally." Speaking of a patient afflicted with this horrid disease, a skilful doctor says: "A banker in Philadelphia died of starvation. He was an inveterate smoker. This habit resulted in impregnating the glands beneath the tongue, which terminated in cancerous ulcerations. Inflammation supervened; the roots of the tongue ulcerated, and the throat sympathized with them until it was difficult to swallow his

spittle. His only nourishment for weeks was of a liquid character; even that, at last, could not be received, and death from starvation and suffocation finally closed the scene, the victim being otherwise in perfect health." The *Medical Times and Gazette* for Oct. 6, 1860, gives an account of 127 cases of cancer of the lip which had been cut out, nearly all of which occurred with smokers. Prof. Bouisson says smoking is the most common cause of cancer in the mouth. An eminent physician some time ago informed us that he never knew one who had ulceration of the mouth who did not either chew or smoke tobacco. Inflamed mouth is also caused by the use of the weed. The Salem *Observer* reports a case of death by cancer in the mouth and throat, caused by excessive smoking. The sufferings of the deceased were most dreadful. At last the cancer, eating into the jugular vein, terminated his life. Dr. Paton, of Paisley, says he has cut out many cancerous affections of the lip, all of which were the result of smoking. An Albany surgeon removed a cancer from a smoker's mouth to save his life. The operation was a very difficult one, and the danger of death from hæmorrhage was very great. The lower lip was divided to a point below the chin, the flaps turned up sufficiently to expose the lower jaw, which was then sawed through at the chin; and after the tongue had been amputated, holes were drilled through the jaw-bone, and it was wired together and the lips replaced. It is also well known that a smoker who has this ulceration of the tongue may give the disease to another by persuading him to use his pipe.

M. Bouisson gives particulars of seventy-two cases of smoker's cancer which he had seen in fourteen years.

The report of the cancer hospital stated " that there had

not been a single case of cancer in the tongue, in that institution, which was not caused by smoking."

Mr. A——, a gentleman about fifty-eight years of age, of a wiry frame and healthy constitution, none of whose relations have ever had a cancerous affection, was observed to articulate with difficulty, his tongue being too large for his mouth. In a short time the tongue had mouldered away—the stump presenting an irregular lumpy surface, covered with a flocculent, dirty, greenish-white deposit. From this to the 2nd of October all his symptoms became aggravated, the salivation more profuse, the perspirations more abundant, and the difficulty of breathing insupportable, and after three hours of intense suffering he expired. "All the death-bed scenes and death-bed sufferings I had ever witnessed," says his medical friend, "were comparatively easy to the individual agonies and gaspings for breath this kind and amiable man was destined to endure." —*Professor Lizars.* So affirm many eminent physicians.

16. *Pulmonary Consumption.*—Several authors of note have recorded instances of consumption caused by tobacco. Says a recent writer of much experience : "To those predisposed to consumption, the ptyalism which tobacco produces hurries on the disease. This is undoubtedly true in many instances. Latent tubercles may sometimes remain undeveloped for a long time, perhaps during the whole natural life of the individual, unless they are roused into action by some acrid and poisonous properties, like tobacco smoke, which tend to irritate and inflame the extremely delicate texture of this important organ, and the result is confirmed and incurable phthisis. The injury to the lungs from hot fumes of tobacco, being so obvious, human ingenuity was long ago put upon the rack to devise means to avoid the mischief without relinquishing the

habit ; this led to the use of the very long pipe, in order to allow the smoke to cool before reaching the lungs ; but the benefit derived from this expedient was found to be trifling, and as the use of such pipes was impracticable in common life, the plan was never extensively adopted, and men chose to ignore the danger rather than relinquish the pernicious practice.   A doctor says that in a large boarding school for young gentlemen, which he professionally attended, the secret habit of smoking indulged in by the elder lads often resulted in incurable consumption, and he quoted one case especially of a bright, clever, and handsome lad, who died at the age of 19, of consumption, brought on by smoking secretly at the tender age of twelve.

17. *Catarrh and Asthma.*—Dr. Perceiro says : " My own observation is unfavorable to the use of tobacco smoke, which I have repeatedly found brings on convulsive cough and spasmodic difficulty of breathing in persons afflicted with chronic catarrh."

A Cheltenham (Eng.) physician once said to a smoking patient, who was suffering from asthma : " I want to keep your lungs quiet, but you irritate them by the fumes of tobacco. You cannot be benefited by medicine if you continue to smoke."

Blatin gives a case of a young officer, whose asthma could be attributed to no other cause, and who was cured by simple abstinence and tonic medicines.

18. *Hypochondria.*—A writer, in giving his own experience, says : " At times I had feelings which seemed to border on mental derangement. I felt that everybody hated me and I, in turn, hated everybody ; I often laid awake nights under the most distressing forebodings ; I have often arisen in fitful and half-delirious slumbers and smoked my pipe to obtain temporary relief from these

sufferings ; I often thought of suicide, but was deterred by a dread of a hereafter. In a few weeks after entirely relinquishing this habit, all these symptoms were gone and my health fully restored."

Dr. Mussey gives a case of a lawyer, who, being accustomed from early life to this stimulant, complained that his life was greatly embittered by incessant and inordinate fear of death. " My spirits," he continues, " were much depressed ; I became exceedingly irresolute, so that it required a great effort to accomplish what I now do without thinking of it ; my sleep was disturbed ; faintings and lassitude were my constant attendants." He gives another case of a man fifty-five years of age, who lost his voice, so as to be unable to speak above a whisper for three years. It is said that "he was subject to fits of extreme melancholy; for whole days he would not speak to anyone ; was exceedingly dyspeptic and subject to nightmare ; he abandoned tobacco, recovered his voice, and his melancholy disappeared."

A medical practitioner in London made the surprising declaration that he had lain awake for hours in the night trembling like a leaf, and feared to look outside his bed curtains lest he should see hobgoblins in his room, and that he never suspected the cause until he heard an anti-tobacco lecture.

19. *Rheumatism.*—It is announced that Senator Carpenter's physician has ordered him to leave Washington for Florida ; his disease, which is called "rheumatism," is said to be largely due to the inordinate use of tobacco. The Milwaukee *Telegram* says : " It is given out that it is rheumatism, but everyone who knows the Senator's habits understands that it is tobacco ; he smokes from twenty to thirty choice cigars a day, and fills in the spare time with pulls at

his pipe; he may go to Florida, but unless he gives up tobacco he will not improve; he is a slave to it, and it is killing him." "Senator Carpenter is a man of more than average intellectual capacity, but he dishonored himself when he consented to become the legal champion of the liquor fraternity; and now, between the alcoholic and tobacco poisoning it appears that he is threatened with utter physical prostration; his unhappy example should serve as a warning to younger men."—*The National Temperance Advocate.*

20. *Other Ailments.*—The half-yearly abstract of the medical sciences for 1854 describes a case of angina pectoris resulting from tobacco using.

Mr. Fenn, of Nayland, Suffolk, England, states that "he has seen very mild cases of typhoid fever rendered fatal from the excessive use of tobacco."

It is authentically stated that the poet Berat was slain at forty-five years of age by that dire disease which is so fell a destroyer of the human race—softening of the brain.

Lauzoni, an Italian author, mentions the case of a tobacco user who fell into a state of somnolency and died lethargic on the tenth day.

An eruption, covering the patient from head to foot, was observed by Dr. Clay, of England; three times it was cured by leaving off snuff, and as often brought on by commencing it.

Nightmare, chronic wakefulness, shocks of the epigastrium, most apt to occur on going to sleep and waking the individual suddenly; on discontinuing tobacco the symptoms vanish.

The following case illustrates how many have their sleep disturbed by the use of tobacco: A sea-captain of more than ordinary good sense was lately asked why he had left off smoking tobacco. He replied: "I had two reasons for it: first, I found that when I smoked I had no appetite for food—I could eat nothing with comfort; but what alarmed me most was that when I went to bed without a cigar a kind of horrors came over me; 1 felt dreadfully and could not go to sleep: would get up and take a cigar and then have a quiet night's rest; I thought if I was so dependent on a foreign stimulant for comfort, it was high time to leave it off; I quit smoking, my appetite returned, is always good, and I can now go to sleep at night more quietly without a cigar than I could formerly with one."

Acne —A pustulous eruption upon the face, which has been known to be excited and kept up by smoking, and to disappear with the discontinuance of the latter.

Hæmoptoe, a spitting up of blood from the throat, Dr. Laycock states is distinctly traceable in some cases to the habit of smoking.

Stricture of the œsophagus—This disease, which in most cases proves fatal, by completely closing the part affected against all food and drink, thus causing that most horrible of all deaths, famishing, Dr. Good asserts has been induced by the use of tobacco.

Depraved appetite—The user of tobacco loses well-nigh all relish for simple and healthful food; he craves continually that which is of the most stimulating and unhealthy kind; pepper, spices, and condiments of every namable variety are consumed by him with avidity.

Depraved thirst—This is one of the worst of the tobacco evils.

Inflamed throat, ulceration of the larynx, fainting fits, cramps in the calves of the legs at night, may be caused by excessive smoking, chewing or snuffing.

Dark greenish hue of the skin, fetid perspiration,

depraved blood, skin disease, foulness of breath from the lungs of the user, pyremia or feverishness, heartburn, gastralgia—a neuralgic affection of the stomach, characterized by pain, often severe, and occurring regularly—water brash, constipation, cramp, or spasm of the stomach, piles or hæmorrhoids, obesity in some cases, spinal weakness, gout, and cephalalgia are caused in many instances by smoking, and sometimes by chewing and snuffing.

Diarrhœa, fistula in ano—a loathsome and often fatal disease—torpor of the liver, malignant disease of the liver, perverted sexuality, impotency, and urinary disorder.

We have now briefly sketched some of the many and dreadful injuries the common use of tobacco does to health, and in view of those pernicious effects is it any wonder that King James I. of England, in 1619, should have characterized tobacco as "loathsome to the eye, hurtful to the nose, harmful to the brain, dangerous to the lungs, and the stinking fumes thereof resemble the horrible Stygian of the pit that is bottomless"?

But what is the fair and logical, as well as scriptural, conclusion the above investigation leads to ?

Clearly this : As life and all the good things we enjoy are the gifts of God, given to us not to trifle with, but to use for the good of our kind and the glory of our Creator, it therefore follows that if the common use of tobacco diminishes blood, muscle, health and strength, as stated above, it must inevitably abridge life, and if so, the habit amounts to suicide in the constructive sense ; hence it is a violation of the sixth commandment, which says, "Thou shalt not kill," and hence a sin.

Says a high authority : "Every man who knowingly brings upon himself disease or death, by tobacco, is a suicide, and drunkards and suicides cannot enter the kingdom of heaven." .

CHAPTER VIII.

TOBACCO USERS MORE LIABLE TO DISEASE.

"There is a way that seemeth right unto a man, but the end thereof are the ways of death."—Prov. xiv. 12.

"As physician to a dispensary in St. Giles during sixteen years, I had extensive opportunities of observing the effects of tobacco upon the health of a very large number of habitual smokers. The extraordinary fact is this: that leeches were killed instantly by the blood of the smokers, so suddenly that they dropped off dead immediately they were applied; and that fleas and bugs, whose bites on the children were as thick as measles, rarely, if ever, attacked the smoking parent. It may be said, 'But why may not the poisonous effect upon leeches, fleas, and bugs be owing to gin, and not tobacco?' The answer to this objection is, that the Arabs and Bedouins, who drink neither wine or strong drink, are protected from the onslaught of the insects which swarm in their tents, by poisoning their blood with tobacco, whilst the wine and spirit drinking Europeans are attacked without mercy."—Extract from an article by J. Pidduck, M.D., in the *Lancet* of the 15th of February, 1856.

Says an English physician: "It is scarcely possible to heal a syphilitic sore, or to unite a fractured bone in a devoted smoker—his constitution seems to be in the same vitiated state as in one afflicted with scurvy." Mr. Fenn, of Suffolk, England, says: "I have seen very mild attacks of typhoid fever rendered fatal from the excessive use of tobacco." Writes another: "During the prevalence of cholera, I have had repeated opportunities of observing that individuals addicted to the use of tobacco, especially those who snuff it, are more disposed to attacks of that disease, and generally in its most malignant and fatal form."

If yellow fever or cholera rages epidemically in a city, the victims of tobacco are among the first to be attacked ; and the chance of recovery among those who use narcotics is always less, other things being equal, than it is with those who are free from such influences, because narcotics are necessarily anti-vital agents.

Pure blood (which tobacco consuming renders impure) resists disease and repels contagion, we are told ; while poisoned blood falls an easy prey. The late Dr. Marshall Hall once said : "The smoker cannot escape the poison of tobacco ; it gets into his blood, travels the whole round of his system, interferes with the heart's action and the general circulation, and affects every organ and fibre of the frame."

"Cigar and snuff manufacturers have come under my care in hospitals, and in private practice ; and such persons cannot recover soon and in a healthy manner from cases of injury or fever. They are more apt to die in epidemics, and more prone to apoplexy and paralysis. The same is true also of those who smoke or chew much."—*Dr. Parker*.

Not only does the use of tobacco render its consumer more liable to disease, but its renunciation has, in many cases, been the cure of a disease—and dire ones, too. The following letter, written to the late Rev. G. Trask, will show this :

" Dear Sir,—I have in mind a young man about twenty-five years old, who was pronounced by his physician to be in a fixed consumption. On calling to see him, I found his room filled with tobacco smoke and he sitting up in bed smoking his pipe; I told him that 'consumptives,' so regarded, had sometimes been cured by dropping tobacco, and begged him to try the experiment.

"His young wife, by a mistaken sympathy, interfered, and said: 'Oh! I wish him to enjoy his pipe and every comfort as long as he lives!' But I persisted, however, and pressed him more and more earnestly to do it.

"A year or two passed away—he had moved out of town—and seeing a neighbor of his, I asked how my young friend was? He told me he was well, was at work at good wages, had a fine little boy, and had perfectly recovered his health. Inquiring for the cure, he said the cure excited some interest; being a slave to tobacco, or his pipe, he had given it up, and consumption with all its attendants had disappeared!"

Dr. Twitchell's "Memoirs," by Dr. Bowditch, published in 1851, reports a case of consumption saved by giving up tobacco; also, a case of nearly fatal nightmare cured by quitting it.

Tobacco renders recovery from disease a greater difficulty.

The Rev. A. F. Gallaway writes: "I have been for some time combating the use of tobacco, as the tap root of intemperance, and one of the most deceiving of sins; for ob, how hard it is for a tobacco devotee to see himself as others see him, and how can he see himself as God sees him! Away here in the South, where I am trying to preach the Gospel, the whole atmosphere is filled with the disgusting stench of tobacco fumes.

"French, Mexicans and negroes are ready to cry out against the man who opposes the use of tobacco, as one who is either insane, puritanical, or enthusiastic. Nothing has afforded us so glad a surprise, and such efficient service, as the sudden appearance of your Anti-Tobacco Books and

Tracts.   Within fifty feet of where I now write, there lives
a poor young man, with a broken leg, a free-born man ! an
abject slave ! enthralled by his despotic master, the pipe !
Thus has he lain for fifty-three days, and no visible sign of
the re-union of the severed bones, unless he can be persuaded to throw away the deadly poison, which has already
reached and diseased his very bone and marrow.   There
he lies, an object of pity, clinging constantly to his idol,
while his mother (a professed Christian) goes about the
house with a pipe almost perpetually fumigating at her
mouth.   Oh, may the God of heaven purify this filthy
nation.   My prayer is, that He may crown with success
every effort you may make in this great work.   I shall do
all in my power to help you.   Your humble brother in
Christ."

Dr. Brewer, who has written upon the effects of tobacco,
mentions the case of a young man, apparently a confirmed
consumptive.   All the usual remedies were applied, but to
no purpose ; he became worse and worse.   At length it
was found that he was continuing to smoke the whole
time ; he was induced to abandon the cigar, and from that
time recovery commenced and proceeded rapidly.

Dr. Cook, a physician of between sixty and seventy
years' practice, whose testimony is entitled to respect upon
this point, asserts : "I am nearly, if not THE oldest medical
practitioner in London, and I have never met with a single
case where it could be said that tobacco smoking had done
good."

"It is an idle excuse," says Dr. R. Martin, "to smoke
tobacco thinking it is good even as a disinfectant to ward
off fevers and epidemics.   Instead of defending the individual against these, tobacco smoking lays him open to
attacks of infectious disease."

" I dispute the alleged benefits of even moderate tobacco smoking as a preventive of damp or malaria ; and serious anomalous symptoms I have seen to arise in the progress of malarious fevers from the abuse of it—such symptoms as may lead to the most grave mistakes in the treatment of fevers, if the medical officer be not careful to inquire into the habits of the patient."—*John Lizars, M.D.*

Dr. R. T. Trall writes : "It has been agreed, even by medical writers, that the habitual use of tobacco is a preventive of bronchitis.   I have seen too many cases of the worst forms of this disease in confirmed tobacco users to credit such closet theory. A similarly superficial observation or reasoning process has induced some medical men to believe that the use of ardent spirits was a preventive of consumption, or the ague and fever.   Although tobacco users, spirit drinkers, and ague and fever subjects do frequently have bronchitis and consumption, it is nevertheless true that these supposed preventives do sometimes obviate one disease by killing the patient with another.   If a man use tobacco enough to waste all his vitality in ten or twenty years, he may die dyspeptic, and so escape bronchitis, as the man who produces an active form of alcoholic disease may die of nervous exhaustion and escape every other ; or the consumptive who gets the ague and fever may die of diseased liver, instead of ulcerated lungs.   It is very true that while the system is possessed of one disease, or occupied with one poison, it is less liable to all other diseases and every other poison, although it is not less liable to death.   This idea of keeping off disease by pre-occupying the system with a poison, or a specific morbid condition, is both nonsensical, unphilosophical, and ridiculously absurd ; health—full, perfect, vigorous, functional integrity, in all

5

the physiological and mental powers—is the only conserva-
tive condition that science knows or nature owns."

"Suppose that it was well established that men who
keep themselves literally soaked in alcohol never had been
known to have dyspepsia, would it prove that this course
of living was judicious? And could it prevent the difficulty by preserving such a uniform healthy action that
dyspepsia could not appear? Certainly not."

Tobacco injures native-born Americans sooner and perhaps more than Germans—those of nervous temperament
and sedentary life quickest, most fatally. There is a won-
derful power in the human stomach to resist and neutralize
the poison of drugs and drinks; some can take opium for
years with apparent impunity. Hungarians eat arsenic
daily, and, as they think, without harm. It is often amid
natural laws as it is under the Divine moral government.
"Because sentence against an evil work is not executed
speedily, therefore the hearts of the sons of men is fully set
in them to do evil."

Nevertheless, it is as sure as fate that all these stimulants
and narcotics derange the organization and sooner or later
strike at the life.

CHAPTER IX.

TOBACCO-USING PARENTS INJURE THEIR OFFSPRING.

" Visiting the iniquity of the fathers upon the children, to the third and fourth generations of them that hate me."—EXOD. xx. 5.

OF all the harm done by the use of tobacco, physically, intellectually, morally and socially, the greatest harm and mightiest wrong done is that of transmitting unto the unborn the appetite for the filthy, unclean, impure, disease creating, misery engendering, taste and desire for smoking, chewing, or snuffing tobacco.

Most strikingly applicable are the words of Ezekiel, ' The fathers have eaten sour grapes, and the children's teeth are set on edge."

" In no instance is the sin of the father more strikingly visited upon his children than the sin of tobacco smoking. The enervation, the hypochondriasis, the hysteria, the insanity, the dwarfish deformities, the consumption, the suffering lives and early deaths of children of inveterate smokers, bear ample testimony to the feebleness and un-soundness of the constitution transmitted by this pernicious habit."—*Dr. Pidduck.*

The following is a medical testimony of no mean authority : " The parent whose blood and secretions are saturated with tobacco, and whose brains and nervous system are semi-narcotized by it, must transmit to his child elements of a distempered body and erratic mind ; a deranged condition of organic atoms, which elevates the

animalism of the future being at the expense of the
intellectual and moral nature." Again, " It could be
shown that the effects of the sins of a heavy smoker upon
his offspring are such that anyone who cared two straws
for anyone besides himself, should abhor the thought of
inflicting an injury upon any living creature, much less
upon the offspring of his body begotten. And here is the
law of hereditary transmission or penalty (Exodus xx. 4,
5, 6), " visiting the iniquity of the fathers upon the children unto the third and fourth generation of them that
hate me." Thus innocent ones are frequently made life-
long sufferers by their drinking, smoking, or licentious
parents. And it is now come to be more widely known
(what is an answer to the apologies of those who indulge
their grosser appetites on the ground that such habits do
not injure themselves) that persons inheriting good constitutions, of laborious life in the open air, will manifest for
years comparatively little conscious injury for their vices,
while children born to them grow up from birth sickly,
weakly, nervous, with the hereditary taints, and sometime
epileptic or imbecile ! And these known 'results might be
inferred from the well-known fact that tobacco chewed is
quickly absorbed into the system from the mouth ; deranges
the action of the heart ; is an energetic depressant of the
nervous system ; while habitual smoking carries the deadly
nicotine through the lungs into arterial blood, depriving
the very springs of life. Were it not that mothers are
generally of purer life and purer blood than fathers, these
deplorable results to offspring would be far more extensively
manifest than now." Excessive smoking has had no small
share in the degeneration of Spain.

"I can point you," says another physician, "to two
families right under my eye, where in each case there is a

nest of little children, rendered idiots by the tobacco habits of their parents!"

"I know a clever man, but an inveterate smoker, who has three sons; the eldest is tall and excessively dull in every way, the second is idiotic, and the third short but of good ability. The youngest is ten years old, and although his parents are still young (about thirty-five), they have never since had a living child."—*Dr. Hampton Brewer.*

Says Mr. Thomas Reynolds: On one occasion I was invited to meet Dr. Browne at an infirmary, and among the patients was a youth about eighteen years of age, suffering from symptoms which I ascribed to tobacco. "What will you say to this case?" said my friend. "This youth has never chewed, smoked, or taken snuff."

"His father did this for him."

"His father! Are you a smoker?" said the Doctor to his father.

"Oh, yes, Dr. Browne."

"How long have you smoked?"

"These five and twenty years."

"Have you," said Dr. Browne, "ever smoked an ounce of tobacco in a day?" "Yes, many times." "This is the iniquity of the father visited on his son," said the Doctor.

Dr. Lazier gives the case of a young lady whose constitution was completely shattered by the smoking habits of her father.

"In a New England town there was formerly a man who had yielded soul and body to the tobacco habit. Rarely was he seen without the pipe or quid. As Johnson said to Boswell, so might a blind man have said of this smoker, "I can't see you, but I smell you." The stench of the pipe was his natural atmosphere. He was able to attend to business, but his offspring were cursed from their birth.

An idiot boy of his would scoop up the loathsome ashes, scraped from his father's pipe, and eat them with avidity! —*Prof. Thwing.*

Sir. B. Brodie writes: "We may here take warning from the fate of the Red Indians of America. An intelligent American physician gives the following explanation of the gradual extinction of this remarkable people: One generation of them became addicted to the use of firewater. They have a degenerate and comparatively imbecile progeny, who indulge in the habit with their parent. Their progeny is still more degenerate; and after a few generations the races cease altogether. We may also take warning from the history of another nation, who, some centuries ago, while following the banners of Soliman the magnificent, were the terror of Christendom, but who since then having become more addicted to tobacco smoking than any of the European nations, are now the lazy and lethargic Turks, held in contempt by all civilized communities."

"The tobacco smoker, especially if he commences the habit early in life and carries it to excess, loses his procreative powers. If he marry he deceives his wife, and disposes her to infidelity, and exposes himself to ignominy and shame. If, however, he should have offspring, they generally are either cut off in infancy, or never reach the period of puberty. His wife is often incapable of having a living child, or she suffers repeated miscarriages, owing to the impotence of her husband. If they have children they are generally stunted in growth or deformed in shape; or incapable of struggling through the diseases incidental to children and die prematurely." Paper published by the British Anti-Tobacco Society.

The following is an extract from a communication in the *Lancet* by Walter Tyrrell, M.R.C.S.:

"More especially would I direct attention to the depressing influence of tobacco on the sexual powers. I feel confident that one of the most common, as well as one of its worst effects, is that of weakening, and in extreme cases, of destroying the generative powers."

Dr. Cleland, in his treatise on the properties, chemical and medical, of tobacco, states that "the circumstance that induced Amurath the Fourth to be strict in punishing tobacco smokers, was the dread he entertained of the population being diminished thereby, from the antaphrodisiac property, which he supposed tobacco to possess."

"How is it, then, that the Eastern nations have not, ere this, become exterminated by a practice which is almost universal? The reply is, that by early marriage before the habit is fully formed or its injurious effects decidedly developed, the evil to the offspring is prevented : but in this country where smoking is commenced early, and marriage is contracted late in life, the evil is entailed in full force upon the offspring." "Against this truth let it not be urged that tobacco users have sometimes comparatively healthy children. So do drunkards. But are they what they could have been, and would have been, had the parent been exempt from all contaminating vices. If there is any one act of criminality which nature stamps with especial abhorrence and punishes with more terrible and relentless severity than all others, it is that of the parent, who by marring his own organization, and vitiating his own functions, bequeaths irremediable physical decrepitude and moral degradation, for the inheritance of his children."

Parents ! The voice of God speaks to you, " Whatsoever you sow that shall you also reap." If then you use tobacco or alcohol, or any other narcotic poison, and transmit to

your children an inherited taste for them, and cultivate
this taste by giving them tea, coffee and spices, as soon as
they are able to sit at your table, look to see the seed you
have planted grow and bear fruit to the unutterable sorrow
to yourselves and eternal ruin to your children. Look to
meet your children and your children's children, at the
judgment day, and have them point the accusing finger at
you, as the cause of their eternal ruin !

Says O. S. Fowler: "Tell me a tobacco chewer is a
virtuous man ? I know better. He may not have broken
the seventh commandment outright ; but as ' he that looketh
on a woman to lust after her committeth adultery with her
in his heart,' so tobacco, in all its forms, causes that sinful,
sensual tone or caste of the love feeling which constitutes
the very essence of licentiousness.

"The influence of tobacco upon amativeness is powerful
and powerfully vitiating. No man can be virtuous as a
companion who uses tobacco ; for although he may not
violate the seventh commandment, yet in the feverish state
of the system which it produces, it necessarily causes a
craving and lustful exercise of amativeness, just as alcoholic
liquors cause such amatory craving ; and for the same
reason. As alcoholic liquors and the grosser forms of
sensuality are twin sisters, so tobacco eating and deviltry
are both one ; because the fierce passions of many tobacco
chewers, as regards the other sex, are immensely increased
by the use of tobacco."

"The stupefying action of tobacco on the system of
generation was one of the phenomena which attracted the
observers at the beginning of its introduction into our intimate habits. In the sixteenth century, it enjoyed a very
great credit in convents, where it was employed under the
name of PRIAPEE, to calm sexual excitement, inherent to

cloister life. It was to be abstained from later, when the disorders it caused in great nervous centres, say, softening, paralysis, and insanity, were perceived.

"Anaphrodisia, or the depression of the genital sense, under the influence of tobacco, comes from two causes: (1) the stupefaction with which narcotism, in general, strikes all nervous centres ; (2) the deleterious action which nicotine has on human germs, which it benumbs or kills as soon as the organism creates them.

"We grow out of a germ, as the wheat grows from a grain; and if any cause whatever, nicotine especially, which is so destructive for all beings, alters the primitive vigor of the human embryo, as the fog would alter the grain inclosed in the wheat, the embryo and the grain, denatured, would give birth but to weak products, and of which the chances of life are quite restrained.

"Here is the true cause of the great mortality of children, before and after birth. Their vigor was faded to the true sources of life by the errors of their fathers in using tobacco.

"The mortality of children has been, for more than a quarter of a century, the great plague of France. Statistics, on the average, show us that half the children coming into the world die in their first year ; before the invasion of tobacco, previous to 1830, death took twenty years to form a similar void.

"In the large cities, Paris, Lyons, Marseilles, where the consumption of tobacco is infinitely more spread than in the country, the mortality of the newly-born is never less than seventy per cent. in their first year."—*H. A. Diepierris, M.D.*

CHAPTER X.

THE USE OF TOBACCO A CURSE TO BOYS AND YOUNG MEN.

"For he that soweth to his flesh shall of the flesh reap corruption."—GAL. vi. 8.

ALMOST everyone believes that the use of tobacco has a blighting effect upon youths. Such is the virulent poison contained in the weed, that when admitted into the stomach of a juvenile, it destroys a most alarming amount of vital force and produces an immediate influence upon his undeveloped system. Look at the fearful effects of smoking and chewing upon the youths of our land! "Their habits are rapidly undermining their health. How many of them are pale and haggard at twenty-one; their cheeks bony, their eyes sunken, their vigor gone, and their whole aspect cadaverous! It seems as if the dreadful savor of the charnel-house had already passed over them!"

Dr. H. V. Miller, of Syracuse, furnishes the following: "A French physician investigated the effects of tobacco smoking upon thirty-eight boys, between the ages of nine and fifteen, who were addicted to the habit. The result was that twenty-three manifested serious derangement of the intellectual faculties, and a strong appetite for alcoholic drinks; three had heart disease; eight, decided deterioration of blood; twelve had frequent nose-bleeding; ten, disturbed sleep; and four, ulceration of the mucous membrane of the mouth."

Says Dr. Waterhouse: "I never observed such pallid faces and so many marks of declining health, nor even knew so many hectical habits and consumptive affections as of late years ; and I trace this alarming inroad on *young constitutions* principally to the pernicious custom of smoking cigars."

Even the *Organ of the Tobacco Trade* admits that " few things could be more pernicious for boys, growing youths and persons of unformed constitutions, than the use of tobacco in any of its forms."

Dr. Richardson remarks that the effects of tobacco "are especially injurious to the youths who are still in the age of adolescence. In these the habit of smoking causes impairment of growth, premature manhood and physical prostration. . . . If a community of youths of both sexes, whose progenitors were finely formed and powerful, were to be trained to the early practice of smoking, and if marriages were to be confined to the smokers, an apparently new and a physically inferior race of men and women would be bred." The poisonous nicotine, which constitutes the active principle of common tobacco, which in a confirmed adult smoker is met and to some extent neutralized by the natural resisting force of the matured human system, lays hold of the forming nerve-tissues of the young, and does its mischievous work unimpeded. Stunted growth, flabby flesh, pasty complexion, shambling gait, fickle appetite, dull comprehension, lack of interest in things, and premature ripeness like that of a diseased apple, are among the signs of injury carried about by thousands of American boy-smokers, who are striving to show themselves men by proving themselves—very foolish children.

The government council of Berne some time ago enacted that young men who are as yet unconfirmed (confirmation is administered in Switzerland between the fifteenth and sixteenth year), are prohibited from using tobacco.

Germany, the paradise of smokers, has adopted stringent measures for the suppression of the habit among boys.

" Let me enter my strongest protest against the abominable custom of youth, at the commencement of puberty, smoking. Boys often think it manly—that is, asserting their manhood—to smoke! Now, this idea is perfectly absurd! Smoking, too, at this particular time, is especially prejudicial; and it has driven many a youth, if he be so predisposed, into a consumption; at other times it has brought on a succession of epileptic fits, which have not only endangered his health, but his very life itself. Stop that boy! A cigar in his mouth, a swagger in his walk, impudence in his face, a care-for-nothingness in his manner. Judging from his demeanor, he is older than his father, wiser than his teacher, and more honored than his master. Stop him; he is going too fast. He does not know his speed. Stop him!—ere tobacco shatters his nerves; ere manly strength gives way to brutish aims and low pursuits. Stop all such boys; they are legion; they bring shame on their families, and become sad and solemn reproaches to themselves."—*H. Chavasse, F.R.C.S.*

At the Edinburgh Reformatory, of eighty boys, there was not one who had not been a smoker or chewer, and most of them had done both. In the reformatory at Blakely, near Manchester, England, out of thirty boys who were admitted soon after its opening, twelve had been smokers, eight chewers, and ten confessed they had stolen tobacco, or money with which to buy it.

An author in the *Medical Gazette*, of Lyons, in treating of smoking by the young, says: "Tobacco smoking lowers the intellectual faculties in a direct manner by its action on the brain, and in an indirect way by predisposing to idleness, and in transforming the natural desire for activity into a desire to remain in a state of inertia. In a moral point of view, it lessens the work of the individual, and relaxes the family ties. The habit becomes associated with evil tendencies, and strengthens them."

Says Dr. A. C. Jackson: "I do not believe there is a boy fourteen years old in the United States, who uses tobacco habitually, who does not also habitually practise self-abuse." Fathers and mothers, who think it will do little or no harm for your sons to use tobacco, ponder on that statement a little.

An almost incredible number of boys are annually *killed* by the deadly poison of tobacco. Dr. Budget, in his treatise on Tobacco, states that in America "it is no uncommon circumstance to hear of inquests on the bodies of smokers, especially youths, the ordinary verdict being, 'died from extreme tobacco smoking.'"

A little child, in the town of L——, picked up a quid and put it into its mouth, thinking it a raisin (a quid that the hired man had thrown upon the floor), and died of the poison during the day.

A boy named West, residing in Swansea, picked up a piece of a cigar in the road, and put it in a pipe and smoked it; in consequence of which he was taken suddenly ill, fell in a state of insensibility, and died in a few hours.

Three young men formed a smoking club, and they all died within two years of the time they formed it. The doctor was asked what they died of. He said they were smoked to death.

"A young man entered Yale College with an athletic frame; but he acquired the habit of using tobacco, and would sit and smoke whole hours together. His friends tried to persuade him to quit the practice ; but he loved his lust, and would have it, live or die—the consequence of which was, he went down to the grave a suicide."—*Prof. Silliman.*

A youth of sixteen dropped dead with a cigar in his mouth. What was the cause ? The coroner's inquest said it was "a mysterious act of God"—an insult to divine goodness. A minister at the funeral repeated the same gratuitous imputation, as if there were no human responsibility in the matter. A sensible lady, who knew the lad's habit, said : "*Tobacco killed him!*"

Dr. Jackson gives a case of a boy who used tobacco so excessively, that he killed himself in a most horrible manner. Before he died, such disorganization of tissue took place as to breed vermin all over his body ; and he expired in the most horrible tortures. The same authority tells of a boy smoker ten years of age, so worn and wasted in flesh, as to be disgusting to look at. As often as twice in twenty-four hours, for more than two years he had epileptic fits, which had ended nearly in the destruction of his intellect. In a fortnight after having been visited by me, he died.

"The sallow complexions, debilitated frames and disordered digestion of the young men of the present day, attest the noxious influence of tobacco ; the plant possesses no salutary qualities ; its use is subversive of all the purely natural functions of life ; impairing the finer sensations of taste, smell and correct feeling."

John Rowland Martin, F.R.S., a great living authority on diseases incident to warm countries, states, from his own observation, that the miseries mental and bodily, produced by cigar smoking, chiefly in young men, far exceed anything detailed in the "Confessions of an Opium-Eater."

Rev. T. L. Kephart says he "attended a session of court

at Doylestown, Penn., at which he witnessed the sad spectacle of a sixteen-year-old boy, the only son of a poor widow, arraigned, tried and convicted of having broken in a pane of glass in the window of a cigar store, and filched therefrom a box of cigars.   Being a smoker, and having no money with which to buy, he resorted to stealing ; and the result was, the widow's son, at that tender age, was doomed to a term either in the house of correction or in the penitentiary—all through smoking."

CHAPTER XI.

TOBACCO THE HANDMAID OF INTEMPERANCE.

"Nor thieves, nor covetous, nor drunkards, nor revilers, nor extortioners, shall inherit the kingdom of God."—1 COR. vi. 10.

IT cannot be questioned that between the habits of tobacco using and drinking there is a close connection, and that the one is very often productive of the other.   If the testimony of some tobacco users and medical men are of any weight, one of the most radical methods of keeping the young from being led to intemperate drinking is to deny them tobacco.   The use of tobacco among boys, says a good old clergyman, is "Satan's seed corn."   Significant name !   The youth who loves the weed will, ten chances to one, make a tippler ; its early habitual use is the training school for drunkenness.

A British physician states that he examined the health of thirty boys, between the ages of nine and fifteen, who were smokers.   In twenty-two of these cases he found various disorders of a serious nature, and more or less marked taste for strong drink—a taste which he found had been generated by tobacco.

The use of this weed is, we think, one of the great attractions to the tavern and parlor of the gin-palace; hence tavern-keepers are always glad to serve their customers with tobacco, and willingly *give* pipes. The blandishments of the rum-seller *draw*, and the insatiable thirst superinduced by tobacco *drives* the poor victim to the cup—" the cup of devils." Tobacco incessantly feeds the appetite for alcohol, and the poor drunkard, attempting to rise, is like a man climbing a perpendicular sand-bank, who comes down as fast as he goes up.

The late Rev. G. Trask asks the following pertinent questions: " Tell us how it is that drunkards are tobacco users, nine to ten—probably ninety-nine to a hundred? Horace Greeley would say, ' Show me a drunkard that don't use tobacco, and we will show you a white blackbird.' Tell us how it is that drunkenness on distilled liquors and this habit were about contemporaneous—began the world together—and, like the Siamese twins, in close bonds and loving style, have come down to us from past generations? Tell us how it is that dram-shops and tobacco-shops are generally identical, or one and the same? Tell us how it is that a dram-shop has a dialect of its own? How is it that poor, drivelling wretches, amidst smoke, saliva and toddy, say as is proverbial, ' I love to smoke because it makes me love to drink, and I love to drink because it makes me love to smoke,' and so on in endless slang? Tell us how it is that our men of science, our reliable physicians, Muzzey, Alcott, Woodward, Agnew, Twitchell, and Warren, Brodie, and a host in Europe, hold it to be a physiological doctrine that one artificial appetite generates another, and that tobacco, by wasting saliva, parching the throat, and inflaming the chest, creates thirst for drink, and paves the way for downright drunkenness? Tell us how it is that a drunkard who merely drops his cups but holds on to his tobacco—often taking the more—has cravings for liquor well-nigh irrepressible; whilst, on the other hand, if he stops his tobacco such cravings are wont to die away? Talk with any poor fellow you see, who has actually passed this ordeal, and he will verify this statement. Tell us how it is that the votaries of tobacco have periodical seasons of depression and goneness, and that multitudes, by confessions, resort to the bottle as an antidote?"

Hence the significant prayer of the Indian, who said, " I wish for three things—first, all the rum there is in the world; secondly, all the tobacco there is in the world; *and*, *then*, more rum!"

"I have no hesitation in averring," says one of the oldest, most able, and experienced temperance advocates (Mr. Joseph Bormond), "that gigantic as are the evils arising from the use of strong drink, those of smoking exceed them."

A well-known temperance advocate writes: "I have known members of the church to break the pledge, but it has nearly always been the case that such have been smokers, and have blamed the pipe for it. So far as I have observed more members of our temperance societies fall from being caught in this snare than in any other."

Another writer says: "The use of tobacco is one of the most powerful accessories of the temptations to drinking which surround British youth." The late Dr. James Hamilton remarked: " Extinguish the pipes of London, and you will go far to shut up the public houses."

It is a fact that in most cases of breach of the Good Templar obligation the man has been a smoker.

The statistics of a whole county of Good Templars showed that the smokers were fully seven times more liable to break their obligation than the non-smokers. Hundreds of the best physicians and temperance workers, both in Europe and America, unite in testifying to the truth of these statements.

In the State's prison in Auburn, N.Y., were six hundred prisoners, confined there for crimes committed when they were under the influence of strong drink; five hundred of them testified that they began their intemperance by the use of tobacco !

According to a manufacturer's recipe, " Opiates, laudanum, and Santa Cruz rum " are among the ingredients used in the making of cigars. One who is familiar with the manufacturing process asserts that tobacco for chewing is thoroughly soaked in a solution of rum and licorice before getting ready for market.

Opium and alcohol, it is said, place their victims in an *abnormal* condition. Tobacco does the same, though in multitudes of cases in a far more thorough and intense degree than alcohol. An inebriate on alcohol may plunge into a debauch to-day and for a while be *abnormal ;* he may, however, emerge to-morrow, and be himself again. The victim of tobacco, it should be said, is in a different condition. He, in some sense, is constantly using it from morning to night. He is thoroughly permeated, and saturated with the insidious and subtle poison. He lives and moves and has his being amidst its nauseous fumigations and saliva, and in strictness of speech, so long as under the power of the poison, he is never in a normal state, and never himself again. Hence the man who is but occasionally drunk on alcohol, is a more hopeful subject of the grace of God than the man who is all the time under the hallucinations of tobacco !

If this is not intemperance, what is intemperance? for does not the Bible clearly define true temperance to be the proper use of good things, total abstinence of bad things?

This intoxication on tobacco can hardly be said to have much distinction from that of the whiskey inebriate. Drunkenness is drunkenness whether effected by alcohol or tobacco ; and " Drunkards shall not inherit the kingdom of God," no matter whether they become such through the influence of spirituous liquors or narcotics. Some—and not a few—smoke themselves to death ; some drink themselves to death ; and which are most guilty, or least guilty, in the sight of God, we are not anxious to determine. We have heard of cases where the lover of the weed—though a professor of religion—has been led into drunkenness, and become a backslider through the use of tobacco. An eminent Baptist minister, in writing on this subject, says : " I have had to exclude from church membership many smokers who have fallen into the sin of intoxication !"

CHAPTER XII.

THE COMMON USE OF TOBACCO A SIN AGAINST SOCIETY.

" Whatsoever ye would that men should do to you, do you even so to them."—MATT. vi. 12.

" SHOULD all other arguments fail to produce a reformation in the conduct of tobacco consumers, there is one which is addressed to good breeding and benevolence, which, for the sake of politeness and humanity, should prevail. Consider how disagreeable your custom is to those who do not follow it, an atmosphere of tobacco effluvia surrounds you wherever you go. Every article about you smells of it; your apartments, your clothes, and even your breath. Nor is there a smell in nature more disagreeable than that of stale tobacco arising in various exhalations from the human body, rendered still more offensive by passing through the pores, and becoming strangely impregnated with the noxious matter which was before insensibly perspired."

" Some of the most disagreeable things relative to the practice against which I have been writing, are still behind the curtain, and designedly detained there; and it is *there alone* where I wish every persevering smoker to seek for a certain vessel named the *spitting dish*, which, to the abuse of all good breeding, and the insult of all delicate feeling, is frequently introduced into public company. May they and their implements, while engaged in this abominable work, be ever kept *out of sight*."—*Dr. A. Clarke.*

" The annoyance and insult to which railway travellers and others are frequently subjected, shows that the acquirement has not mended their manners. The very presence of heavy smokers in a crowded and heated assembly, with nature at work to expel the nicotine from their insulted bodies, makes the whole company suffer from the loathsome nuisance. Smokers are (most of them) selfish and disagreeable, they have but little regard for the comfort of others. They have only to remember their own unpleasant feelings when learning to smoke to be convinced how disgusting the weed is to those who do not use it ; yet the average smoker will puff his abominable fumes under your very nose, with an air of indifference as sublime as if he were diffusing the aroma of roses."

" The unseemly pipe and cigar, the sucking and pulling, the selfish insolence of the smoker in forcing the poisonous smoke, after having been in his dirty mouth and diseased lungs, into the clothes, food and drink, into the apartments, faces, mouths and lungs of clean persons, ladies and children especially, may be fashionable, but, to say the least, it is not in harmony with the golden rule thus to insult society. Why are these sickening presentations viewed with so little manifestation of disgust, even by the refined ? Mostly because we are used to them—they are popular and fashionable."

> " Vice is a monster of so frightful mien,
> That to be hated needs but to be seen ;
> But seen too oft familiar with her face,
> We first endure, then pity, then embrace."

" How sensible men can feel comfortable while seeing those with whom they are conversing avert their faces— turn from their disgusting breath—we do not know. Can it be, that those who use the filthy weed think that they are making themselves a nuisance for the glory of God !

Such people must know, that they are slaves to a foolish, debasing lust, which has greater influence over them than their respect for their neighbors' comfort, or regard for the claims of God.

"Some respect should be had in our *eating* and *drinking* to the comfort, safety and convenience of others. No man has a right to drink what will take away his senses, and render him a terror or disgrace to his friends. No true man (not to say Christian) will do this, who has any proper regard for the rights of his fellowmen. I know not how anyone can be justified who makes his *person* or his *breath* nauseating and disgusting to all who meet him. 'If any man defile the temple of God, which temple ye are, *him will God destroy.*'

"Why are not these unclean persons put aside from society for the same reason that dead animals are removed from the sidewalks in our cities?

"Besides our every-day experience shows us that the pipe *divides* instead of *uniting* society. In company the smoker is an abomination, who must be turned into a *separate* room. He must seek a retreat in some obscure nook, where his nauseous fumes will not offend the nostrils of the other members of the party. And when he returns from his banishment to the general circle the stench that he brings with him makes many keep at a distance from him. And yet, if compelled to pass a whole afternoon and evening *without* a pipe or quid, he would be moody and restless, and one would be scarcely able to get a civil answer from him!"

"'Do thyself no harm,' is an important precept in moral science; and no man can habitually imbibe the poisonous fumes of tobacco without harm. Therefore, if we observe the moral law, we have not a right to smoke. But we

know you will smoke ; so, assuming that, we wish kindly
to point out to you some things you have no right to do.

" First, you have no right to smoke in your own home,
or any home, where there are women and children. The
lady of the house may very generously inform you that the
smoke is not disagreeable to her, but that does not make it
right for you to smoke in her presence. Tobacco contains
an active poison, and there are particles of this poison
floated off in the smoke, to be breathed by the inmates of
the house. You will agree with me that it would not be
right for you to bring arsenic in the house, and allow
women and children to be poisoned by the fumes. The
same principles apply to the poison of tobacco. We have
seen cases reported by physicians, where delicate children
have died from the tobacco poison floating in the air of the
home. If you will poison yourself, you have no right to
poison the air for others. Besides this, if your boys survive
the poisoning when they are babes, and grow up, they will
become so saturated with tobacco that they will be likely
to grow up smokers. You have no right thus to perpetuate
a bad habit.

"On the same principle you have no right to smoke in
stores or public offices, or any other room into which women
and children are likely to come. Neither have you a right
to saturate your breath or your garments with tobacco
smoke, and then go to your home or into a public assembly.
If you must smoke, you should change your garments and
sweeten your breath before you go into society. Men
recognize this principle on the cars, and smoke in the
smoking-car. Why not always regard it in society? But
you say, If I cannot smoke in the house you will not allow
me the right of smoking on the street. Yes, if you will go
into a street where no one else will go. But if you smoke

on the street corners, or walk along the sidewalk puffing your cigar, there are hundreds of others whose business requires them to walk there, too. Some of these are nauseated with tobacco, and others will inhale the poisonous smoke and be injured by it.

"Besides this, the effect of loading the air with smoke, and yourself setting the example, which in the home would tend to make your own boys smokers, on the streets will make your neighbors' boys smokers. We would say, then, that, consistently with the right of others, you have no right to smoke on the public streets.

"But do you ask, Where shall I smoke? We answer, if you will smoke, go into the fields by yourself, or else have a room into which none but smokers will have occasion to go; have it in the attic, if possible, so that the poison may be dissipated, and not injure others. Have a cap and coat to put on while smoking, so as not to saturate the clothes which you wear in the company of others. In this way you can 'enjoy' your pipe, and not infringe upon the rights of others.

"Smokers have rights which we are glad to respect, and others have a right to walk the streets, or enter stores or public places, or to sit down in our homes, without having the air poisoned by tobacco."—*Informer.*

" Witness, too, the effect upon the feelings, when by accident or otherwise, a man is deprived of his tobacco. He becomes unhappy, irritable and snappish even to his wife and children—those to whom he should above all others be kind.

"Wherever we go we are reminded that smoking is the foe of good fellowship. In places of public amusement, how often does the announcement, ' No smoking allowed !' meet the eye. On some railways they provide cars for the

principal trains, into which the smokers may be turned as
sheep into a pen, and such cars are labelled ' For smokers.'
Thus everywhere the poor smoker goes about, Cain-like,
with the brand of 'a pest to society' written on his brow."

"To those who make the objection—'But this is a free
country, and have I not the right to smoke?' we answer,
yes, Mr. Smoker, this is a free country, and other people
have rights as well as you; and so you have not a right to
annoy others unnecessarily."

Smokers had better follow the example of the Duke of
Norfolk, who has a smoking-room over the upper stories of
a quadrangular tower seventy feet high.

CHAPTER XIII.

DOES THE TOBACCO HABIT GLORIFY GOD?

"Whether therefore ye eat or drink, or whatsoever ye do, do
all to the glory of God."—1 COR. x. 31.

It is very evident that God has created man for a great
and noble end,—the glory of himself. Man is expected
and commanded to make everything he does subserve to
this end. He must neither eat nor drink, nor do *anything*
that will not be for the glory of God. In short, it must
be the one ruling motive of his life to please the Lord.
How clearly and strongly is the common use of the weed
condemned by this rule! Can the habitual use of a drug
so deleterious in its effects upon the human frame, so
injurious to the soul, and the handmaid of drunkenness—
be conducive to the glory of God? Never—no never!

Who will dare to say that the puffing and blowing, the spitting and chewing of tobacco users, together with the time lost and money squandered, health injured, and bad example set, are for the glory of God?

How can any person, for the glory of God, create appetites and lusts for filthy, useless and injurious weeds, drugs and drinks, when he knows that these lusts, once formed, will have greater power over him than any other? "Know ye not, that to whom ye yield yourselves servants to obey, his servants ye are whom ye obey?"

How can any Christian, having formed such appetites, continue in subjection to them to the glory of God? "Let not sin, therefore, reign in your mortal body, that ye should obey it in the lusts thereof."

There can be no *utility* nor *virtue* in using nauseating and disgusting substances and drinks for which we have no natural taste, till we create artificial hankering for them, which actually enslaves for life nearly every person who becomes a subject to it. "They that are Christ's, have *crucified the flesh with the affections and lusts.*"

Can a Christian with impunity, by practice and example, lure others on into like filthy, expensive, unhealthy bondage? "Ye are the light of the world." He is a carnal man who does so, even though he is a minister. He by no means seeks to "do all to the glory of God."

Does it glorify God to fill the air with poisonous smoke and vapors for others to breathe, or to spit tobacco juice about for decent people to look at and walk in? We read of some, "whose God is their belly, whose glory is in their shame, and whose end is destruction."

What tobacco devotee who loves the Lord would like, before lighting his pipe or cigar, to get down on his knees, and beseech Heaven to bless the weed to the good of his body, and the glory of God? Would he like to say, Lord, let the consumption of this tobacco into smoke, or a piece of useless, filthy quid, be acceptable to thee, and nourish my body? I think there are but few, even of the most confirmed tobacco users, who would feel like doing such a preposterous and wicked thing. Yet no man is at liberty to consume anything upon which he cannot ask God's blessing, and which he knows will not be for his glory. It is utter folly to argue that because there is no passage in the Bible that says, "Thou shalt not use tobacco," that therefore it is lawful to use it. The Bible is essentially a book of principles : and it is left to common sense and honesty to apply those principles. In the passage which begins this chapter, we have a clear and safe guiding principle for every circumstance and condition of life. It is too plain to be misunderstood : it bears right on the subject in question. Surely, if we wish to be led by Bible teaching at all, we shall not, in the very face of this principle—which is tantamount to a direct command—complain that the Scriptures say nothing against the use of tobacco.

CHAPTER XIV.

THE EXAMPLE OF SMOKING AND CHEWING PERNICIOUS.

"Let your light so shine before men, that they may see your good works and glorify your Father which is in heaven."—MATT. v. 16.

THAT the example of smoking and chewing is most pernicious and contagious but very few will be found to deny. A prison investigation once showed, that out of 700 male convicts then there, 600 were committed for crime done under the influence of liquor; that 500 out of the 600 testified tobacco smoking was the beginning of their intemperance.   This fact alone shows what a fearful responsibility there is in a smoker's example; yet it is a sad truth that this idle, useless habit, has in the majority of cases been copied from the example of some adult who was, perhaps, a professor of religion.

The acknowledged banefulness of the weed by devotees of tobacco themselves, is additional proof that their example cannot but be an evil one; and, moreover, they would feel an *uneasiness* in learning their sons to smoke.

"Who would not be shocked to learn that all the little children in the land, from five to ten years old, had commenced smoking cigars, etc., in perfect imitation of their older people?

"Suppose our mothers, wives, sisters and daughters should commence to smoke cigars and meerschaums, to chew and spit, and imitate all the tobacco airs of tobacco-using males, privately and publicly! Who would think them any neater, more attractive, or lovable, for these acquirements?"

"Your moral sense revolts from the spectacle of smoking boys and youths. But why should it, if smoking be a *harmless pleasure?* Some of you are parents, and feel that you would rather do anything than encourage your children to grow up confirmed smokers. But why should you feel so anxious that your children should not become thorough devotees of the weed, if you are perfectly sure that *you* are in the path of duty by using it so freely? Can you be doing right by cherishing a habit in which you would not like your children to imitate you? Let the voice of conscience speak, and be sure that *a practice which you feel you could not innocently teach your own sons cannot be innocently indulged by yourself.*"

Here is a case to the point given by Rev. G. Trask: "To show how important is *example* in the matter, I may mention that a few Sundays ago, on speaking seriously to a half-clad lad belonging to our school, on the folly of his practice, he very quickly turned upon me with '*why, some of the teachers smoke.*'

"I replied, 'I should think not. What makes you think they do?' 'Because I seed one on 'em (at the same time describing him), one day, go into a cigar shop, an' buy a cigar.'

"'But very probably you were mistaken; for the other day I myself was in a public house on business, and when I came out there stood, at a little distance off, two of our lads, who, if they saw me, would probably think I had been drinking, but I had not. Indeed, I was so fearful lest they should think so, and be injured by my example, that I felt much inclined to go and tell them I had not.' With an arch and confident look, the boy replied, 'O no,

I wasn't mistaken; for I stood and watched him, and seed him come out wi' it lighted in his mouth; and I think he seed me too, for he turned his head another way and looked stylish.'"

Dear Christian brother who may read these pages, perhaps you are engaged in some work for the Master; consider your position. Having espoused the cause of Christ, and given yourself to Him, you are a spectacle to men and angels; companions see you smoke, and they smoke, you endorse the lust, and confirm them in sin. Away with this stumbling-block, which causes your brother to stumble.

CHAPTER XV.

FACTS FOR TOBACCO-USING MINISTERS.

" Be ye clean that bear the vessels of the Lord."—Isa. lii. 2.

WITH what consistency can smoking ministers condemn other physical and moral uncleanness without condemning tobacco? But are not many led into the practice of smoking by the example of their pastors? With profound grief we have to answer, yes.

Thousands of little boys—*puny, sickly, nervous* little boys—in our cities are chewing, spitting and smoking every old stub of tobacco they can pick up, or anything resembling it. When their parents or minister chew or smoke, it helps them amazingly.

A writer in a New York paper mentions how he was astounded at a conference of ministers, to see at the house of a friend, where the ministers were entertained, a spittoon of the largest kind, overflowing with the united expectorations of one bishop, two presiding elders, three ministers and one preacher on trial.

Imagine a minister known as a smoker, or as a snuff-taker ; or, suppose one addicted to chewing tobacco, should enter the pulpit, having a quid of the fetid weed in his mouth. What effect would his preaching have on a morally enlightened and common sense congregation, were he to preach from the text : " Abstain from fleshly lusts which war against the soul ?"

Most tobacco-using ministers would be astonished, if they knew to how many in their congregations, their stench of person renders them offensive ; how many house-keepers open their doors and windows, to air their rooms after their pastor's social call ; how many persons shrink from the nauseating odors of the tobacco-perfumed study, when desiring religious counsel. For, be it remembered, that it is not his person alone which the use of tobacco renders offensive ; his smoking-room, and his whole house suffers similarly. Curtains, carpet, furniture, pictures and books, all reek alike with the foul residuum of stale tobacco smoke. There is no such thing as a clean room where tobacco is used. Said a gentleman recently : " I had a smoking clergyman at my house for some weeks. He smoked in the room which he used as a study ; he has been away from us now five months. We have done everything in our power to cleanse that room ; but on a damp day when the air is heavy, the smell of old tobacco smoke is distinctly perceptible there."

How would Paul and Peter and John look, standing up now among the people in the house of God, with quids of tobacco in their mouths, with its juices defiling their lips, spitting the stuff in every direction; spending ten or twenty dollars of their stinted salary every year on this besotting, enslaving sin, and preaching the doctrine of self-denial, crucifixion of the flesh, pecuniary economy and liberal support of the Lord's treasury?

One man said he knew ministers who could get along better without prayer than go one day without tobacco. Shall ministers be a party to this robbery of God's treasury?

"I am sorry to have it to say, that this idle, disgraceful habit prevails much at present among ministers of most denominations. Can such persons preach against self-indulgence, destruction of time or waste of money? These men greatly injure their own usefulness; they smoke away their own ministerial importance in the families where they visit; the very children and maidservants pass their jokes on the 'piping parson,' and should they succeed in bringing over the uninfected to their vile custom, the evil is doubled. I have known serious misunderstandings produced in certain families in which the example of the idle parson has led to such a calamity. Some are so brought under the power of this disgraceful habit, that they must have their pipe immediately before they enter the pulpit. What a preparation for announcing the righteousness of God, and preaching the Gospel of the Lord Jesus Christ? Did St. Paul do anything like this? No, you say, 'for he had the inspiration of the Holy Spirit.' Then you take it to supply the place of this inspiration! How can such persons smile at their own conduct? 'Be ye followers of us as we are of Christ Jesus,' can never proceed out of their lips."—*Dr. Adam Clarke.*

How can the Christian minister stand up before the people, and from the sacred desk proclaim the beauty of holiness, while he is known to be the abject slave of a disgusting and ungentlemanly habit? How can he lead sinners to forsake the world, the flesh, and the devil, when he is not himself an example of common decency? How can he exhort and pray in the conference meeting and at the family altar, when his breath is offensive to all whom he approaches?

"Ministers are to be an example to the believers. (1 Tim. iv. 12.) They are to present to their flocks, and especially to their young people, a living and a practical illustration of all the Christian virtues. Now, suppose a case: You are invited to dine with one of your people who has a son, a 'fast young man,' a terrible smoker of cigars, and a great grief to his parents. *Smoking is one of the things that is ruining him.* But he sees *you* smoke and you confirm him in the habit! The next time his afflicted father reasons with him on the necessity of abandoning the practice, he is met by a quotation of *your* example, and is coolly told that his *own pastor smokes.'* It is a fearful thing when they who have "to watch for souls," become the means of *confirming souls in sin.* But, certainly, a pastor who is an inveterate smoker must do *some* injury, in some few quarters, *to say the least,* by his devotion to this habit. I believe, however, that the greater part of the injury which such a man does, is done *quietly* and *secretly even to himself.* He will never know all the mischief he has occasioned until, at the last great day, he is confronted with it at the bar of God. For the influence of ministers steals into the houses of their flock, and permeates the families dwelling there, and radiates through the locality in which they labor; so that thousands are every moment more or less affected by their lives. If the salvation of souls is our one great object, ought we not to be willing to forego any and every such *questionable*

7

habit—to use no stronger phrase—as smoking, rather than
add to the jeopardy in which *a single soul* is placed?
Anything rather than imperil the salvation of a fellow-
creature! Anything rather than raise a barrier in the
way of the reception of our message by *a solitary hearer.'*
And my own experience enables me to say, *with perfect
confidence*, that no minister of the Gospel can be addicted
to tobacco without injuring his usefulness in some quarter.
Will my honored brethren, then, who still smoke, bear
with me, if I ask them to look this fact fairly in the face?
Sure I am that they ought to decide, once and forever, to
abandon the habit. Anything that can enfeeble the strain
of a minister's address when speaking to such characters
(young smokers); anything that can take off the edge of
his warning and expostulations, should be carefully avoided.
And I feel that, now I touch neither pipe nor cigar myself,
I am in a much better position for dealing with such cases
than I formerly was. No youth who wastes his shillings
a week on cigars, or other things to which cigar-smoking
generally leads, can turn on me now and say: 'Physician,
heal thyself.' "—*From " Confessions of an Old Smoker."*

It has been truly said, that evil habits in good men
work, by their example, immeasurably more harm than
evil habits in bad men. Hence the holy apostle's injunction : "Nor *anything* whereby thy brother stumbleth, or
is offended, or is made *weak.*" Yet see the ministers and
the deacons working their devoted tobacco mills, week-
days and Sundays. They sit down to their strip of the
solid plug, and begin to bite and chew, and chew and spit;
and they go on biting and chewing, and praying and
spewing without cessation, year in and year out : till by
uncommon Christian faithfulness in the course of fifty
years—if they should live so long to bless and bedaub the

world—they have finished their strip of one or two miles' length!

Bishop Ames, of the Methodist Episcopal Church, once declared before the New England Annual Conference, that it was his solemn conviction that a large portion of the funds for superannuated preachers is paid to men mentally and physically disqualified by the use of tobacco.

An eminent minister said he was walking the streets of Rochester, N.Y., -the place of his residence—with a lighted cigar in his mouth, as the better class of loafers would do, when an avowed infidel of his acquaintance met him, and instantly burst into a fit of laughter. The preacher, wishing to know what pleased him so, was answered with: "Oh! I was thinking how you would look going up to meet the Lord amid wreaths of tobacco smoke, with that cigar in your mouth!" The minister abandoned the weed.

How sad it is for a minister to be turned away from a death-bed, on account of the stench of tobacco on him! Yet, dear saints in the agonies of death have, with pale and trembling hand, waved tobacco-using pastors from their bedsides—pastors they loved!

CHAPTER XVI.

THE COMMON USE OF TOBACCO A DIRECT CURSE TO THE SOUL.

"Quench not the Spirit."—1 Thess. v. 19.

WE sometimes hear the question asked, "What has tobacco to do with religion?" The common use of this weed is a violation of the revealed will of God. Though the Bible does not mention this habit by name, yet "the commandment is exceeding broad," so as to cover many acts and practices which, to an enlightened conscience, are *sins*, although not specified in the Decalogue. This habit is also a violation of the laws of nature. And, be it remembered, a crime against nature is a crime against God. A crime against divine law written in God's book of nature, in which He reveals His will, may be as fearful in magnitude as a crime against divine law written in the Bible.

A long and careful observation of the effects of tobacco habits has convinced us that the common use of the weed is a direct curse to the souls of men, and is a fearful hindrance to the spread of Christianity. As evidence of this, see prison statistics. *With scarcely an exception, forgers, defaulters, and swindlers use tobacco;* while 97 per cent. of all male convicts first lose their freedom by the bondage of tobacco.

Speaking of the decay of the senses caused by tobacco, the *Scalpel* says : " If there is a vice more prostrating to the body and mind, and more crucifying to all the sympathies of man's spiritual nature, we have yet to be convinced of it."

Tobacco using, even more than liquor drinking, disqualifies the mind for exercising its intuitions concerning the right and wrong; it degrades the moral sense below the intellectual recognitions.

A New York physician writes: "The universal experience of all mankind will attest, and the intelligent observation of every individual will confirm the statement, that precisely in the ratio that persons indulge in narcotic stimulants, the mental powers are unbalanced, the lower propensities acquiring undue and inordinate activity at the expense, not only of the vital stamina, but also at the expense of the intellectual and moral nature. The whole being is not only perverted, but introverted and retroverted. The association of tobacco and alcohol with gambling, prostitution and all the disreputable avocations in society is sufficient attestation of this principle. Those who can understand the easy transition from foul blood, disturbed circulation, and preternatural excitement of the animal passions, to immoral conduct and general licentiousness, will not wonder at the frequent and otherwise unaccountable eccentricities, debaucheries, or even crimes of men in high positions.

Tobacco leaves its apathetic victims an easy prey to temptation. It often induces habits of indolence, apathy, and inactivity; leads its victims into bad associations, and produces morbid excitability and irritability. It leads to forgetfulness of God and the duty of self-denial. It begets strife in the railway car and temperance house. Being much in demand, induces many to keep open their stores on Sabbath. It keeps many away from the house of God and the Sabbath school.

Tobacco is praised as a soporific—as a comfort and solace in trouble. Yes, here is the world-wide mischief of this narcotic. Thousands of young and old men hear the Gospel preached, are awakened, resolve to become Christians, thank God for a good cigar which allays their fears, and quiets their disturbed mind. We have every reason to believe that thousands of awakened souls have been lulled to sleep again by the use of the stupefying drug.

A professor of religion and a slave of tobacco may mean well; but a hallucination pervades his moral nature exactly proportioned to the amount of tobacco he consumes. He may have an intellectual consciousness of right and wrong, but the moral sense is blunted; he does not *feel* duty if he sees it; nor does he *feel* truth as he perceives it.

Multitudes can testify to the awful truth of these statements; and if space permitted we might give hundreds of facts in proof of what we have laid down; but a few must suffice. Says an old smoker: "Tobacco smoke deadens sensibility and fills the soul with self-satisfaction. The smoker, whilst sublimely fumigating earth and air, is satisfied! He is satisfied, whether rich or poor, married or single, *if he has a pipe!* He is satisfied whether in the forecastle or cabin, whether at the head of a factory or an understrapper, *if he has a pipe!* He is satisfied, whether he knows much or little, whether saint or sinner, *if he has a pipe!*"

Here is another—but sad confession: "I was at church, when fidelity to my idol would allow; and often was I moved with ideas of 'wrath to come,' and hurried home to drown in tobacco fumes the strivings of God's Spirit. Often have I writhed under mighty truths from Sinai and Calvary; often has my meerschaum, like the bacchanalian cup, relieved every twinge of pain and every fear."

A deacon once said, in self-defence against an appeal to his conscience, on the subject of using tobacco, " If I go to conference or prayer meeting without first smoking, or taking a chew of tobacco with me, I cannot enjoy the meeting : I cannot speak or pray without it; the meeting passes like a dull and heavy task ; I enjoy none of its exercises, and long to have it close, that I may procure relief. But when I previously smoke, or carry my plug of tobacco with me, I then can enjoy the meeting —can talk and pray, get good, and do good, and all goes well."

The reply in substance was this :   " Instead, deacon, of going to the social meeting, under the inspiration of the Holy Ghost, depending on His agency to give you enjoyment, and freedom of feeling, and utterance, you go there leaning on the inspiration of tobacco—an agency not from above—one that is earthly, sensual, devilish."

This is a perfect sample of the condition and feeling of thousands—and more or less of all tobacco users.   They so deaden the natural sensibilities of body and mind by using it, that they are not immediately susceptible of the impulses of the Holy Spirit, by which alone a true spirit of devotion and religious enjoyment is induced.   Everything to them is insipid and lifeless without their tobacco.   They absolutely depend on its exciting properties to give them what they call spiritual life !

Writes a friend : " A young man, of my acquaintance, between twenty-five and thirty, became very sick ; he was irreligious and profane, and a neglector of the Word of God. I felt it to be my duty to visit him in his sickness ; hence called at his residence, and was admitted to his bed-side.   I conversed with him a few moments, directing him to the blessed Saviour Jesus Christ, whose blood cleanseth from all sin.   He made no reply, but called immediately for his *pipe*, and beckoned me to leave. I moved round to the opposite side of his bed, and while lying on his back *smoking*, his head a little raised, I asked him if he suffered much pain? He immediately replied in a firm voice, 'Your conversation gives me more pain than anything else!'" This is an illustration of the repeated fact, that the use of tobacco abases, stupefies, and quiets conscience, and endangers the souls of its victims.

The late Rev. George Trask thus cogently writes: "Account for the mournful fact if you can, that a drug so nauseous, in spite of every taste and every instinct, now has mastery over *two hundred millions*, without the hypothesis that Satan has a hand in it! Render unto Satan the things that are Satan's.

"Tobacco stupefies sensibility, produces self-satisfaction, and soothes the subjects of Satan in their sins? Its lulling potency makes many a minister an amiable dolt; robs him of zeal for *Revivals*, and of courage to wield the battle-axe; seats him in his easy-chair to nurse his dignity, and to be satisfied with his spiritual attainments, till death winds up the scene!

"Tobacco to thousands of young men has unearthly charms. It allays anxiety, extracts arrows of conviction, and makes them satisfied whether saints or sinners. It not only renders them insensible to the Gospel, but it often *paralyzes the will*; and its victim is like a fort, with traitors within and enemies without, while the sentinel is drunk! It often breaks down all *manliness*; and the victim is in the condition of the poor collegian, who in tears cried, 'what I would that I do not, but what I hate that I do.' '*Oh, I need tobacco to give me resolution to give up tobacco.*'

"It is deplorable enough that the Gospel must encounter

a heart which is at enmity with God ; but oh, if it must encounter not only an enemy but a sot ; not only a sot, but a paralytic ; not only a paralytic, but a fool—the case is incomparably worse.

"Such are the effects of tobacco, *not on all*, but on multitudes who hear the Gospel. Satan knows this ; and, if he does not, he has not the sagacity commonly ascribed to him, and he is unfit for his office."

The following dream relates to an old lady, who was professedly very pious, but, like thousands in the Church, for many years allowed her devotions to her pipe to exceed her devotions to God. She was more sure not to forget her vows to this carnal appetite, than not to forget her closet for prayer. One night she dreamed of an aerial flight to the regions of the spirit-world, where not only her eyes could feast on the beauties of elysian fields, but where she could converse with perfected spirits. She asked one of these to go and look for her name in the Book of Life. He complied ; but at length returned, with a sad countenance, saying it was not there. Again she besought him to go, and search more thoroughly. After a more lengthy examination, he returned without finding it. She wept bitterly, and could not rest till a third search should be made. After a long and anxious absence the messenger returned, with a brightened countenance, saying that it had, after great labor, been found ; but that, so deep was the covering which years of tobacco smoke had laid over it, it was with great difficulty that it could be discerned. She awoke, and found herself prostrated with weeping. It is not for me to say whether there was, or was not, any divine instruction in this dream ; but it produced in the old lady repentance, and a pious resolution henceforward to give unto God, not a divided, but a whole heart,—to cast the idol at her feet, and lay no more of her time, money, and vital energies upon its unholy altar.—*Sel.*

We will close this chapter with the following striking letter which we received some years ago :

"DEAR BRO.,—It is inexpressible how devoted some people are to the quid, the pipe, and the vile stuff they call snuff. Never did a child eat poundcake or candy with a greater relish than they manifest in masticating their filthy quids, smoking their miserable black pipes, or shovelling up their noses that nasty snuff, that renders their utterances so thick and indistinct, that no one can understand a word they say, until, after having buried their faces in their handkerchiefs, and, by repeated blasts as loud as any horn, they clear their heads, in order to be able to hold intelligent conversation. Oh, that men would be persuaded to throw away their tobacco boxes, break their pipes, and forswear the nauseous weed forever !

" In a place where we were stationed some few years ago, we had a local preacher who was an ardent tobacco devotee. One evening, being late home from work, he hurriedly washed, took his supper and started out to meeting. In starting out, however, he placed in his mouth the inevitable quid. When he arrived at the meeting, he found there was no one to take charge. The hymn book was immediately placed in his hand, with the request that he would open the meeting. He announced a hymn, which was spiritedly sung by the congregation. The influence of the Spirit was present, and was soon manifested in the responses of the congregation. The man felt happy, and, forgetting the miserable black intruder he had in his mouth, he prayed with all his might, his throat distended like 'an open sepulchre,' and the black occupant of his mouth slid down to its tomb. Then, oh ! gulph, heave, cough, spit—bringing his prayer to an abrupt termination. The thought passed through his mind as swift as lightning, 'serve the Lord with clean lips,' his conscience stung him to the quick, and he resolved never to use tobacco again."

" We believe this book, 'The Common Use of Tobacco,' is calculated to do great good.   That it has done good we are already assured.   One person, to whom we gave a copy, told us that his brother-in-law, to whom he had lent the book (and who was an inveterate user of tobacco), had been so thoroughly convinced of the evil by a perusal of the pamphlet, that he had given up the practice altogether."

CHAPTER XVII.

THE TIME WASTED IN THE INDULGENCE OF TOBACCO.

" Redeeming the time."—Eph. v. 16.

"THE loss of time in this shameful work is a serious evil.   I have known some who, strange to tell, have smoked three or four hours a day by their own confessions ; and others who have spent six hours in the same employment.   How can such persons answer for this at the bar of God."—Dr. A. Clarke.

Says the Scientific American : "A correspondent recently timed the smokes taken in a day by twelve journeymen painters, who were engaged on a job requiring special haste. The total number of minutes footed up over a quarter of a day's work, and the employer soon discovered that he could not afford any such loss, and promptly forbade the practice."

The aggregation of time—which is said to be money—lost by the smoking community, is out of the reach of computation. A puffer acknowledges that twenty minutes are required to smoke a pipe or cigar. Take the average of three per day. Thus, at the end of twelve years, one whole year has been wasted—worse than wasted. Is not this also an encouragement of idleness?

Lord Stanhope calculated that in forty years, two years were dedicated by a snuffer to tickling his nose, and two to blowing it. A generous smoker will devote a much larger proportion of time than this to his cigar or pipe. But that is a trifle compared with the sacrifice of time which grows out of the bodily indolence and the aversion of intellectual activity begotten by the habit. Multiply this by the whole number of tobacco users, and it will amount to centuries of precious time consumed in useless practices.

Says a writer : " I once crossed the Atlantic with a venerable sea-captain, who had been a snuffer of tobacco for about fifty years. One of the passengers had the curiosity to ascertain the time he had consumed in the operation of taking the pulverized poison. Much to the amusement of the passengers, and the mortification of the captain, it appeared that more than one year of the time allotted to him by his Maker had been occupied in plying his thumb and finger in supplying his nasal cavity with this odoriferous powder, and in taking care of the disgusting drippings it expelled from his nose, which had grown to the form of a knurly pink-eyed potato, from the lengthened abuse of that organ ! "

We might calculate the time spent in *taking a chew or lighting a cigar*, and prove that it would be sufficient, if rightly spent, to give the man a knowledge of several sciences ; but at present we will push our calculations no further. " The time is short." (1 Cor. vii. 29.)

CHAPTER XVIII.

TOBACCO A DESTROYER OF PROPERTY.

"Wasting and destruction are in their paths."—ISA. lix. 7.

THE mere waste of money is not the only disaster resulting from the use of tobacco.   Thousands upon thousands
of the most destructive fires and many deaths have been
caused by sparks from tobacco pipes.

Mr. Braddely stated in his report for 1860, that "fifty-
three of the fires of the English metropolis had been traced
to the carelessness of smokers in throwing away the burning ends of cigars."

In a single fire at San Francisco a few years ago, caused
by carelessness in the use of a cigar, several millions of
dollars' worth of property were destroyed.

In a destructive fire at Boston some time ago caused by
a pipe, eight men perished in the flames.

"'A smoker in smoking ceases to think,' says a French
writer, and the recklessness with which firebrands are
carried about the streets, stores and ships, or among com-
bustible merchandise, seems to verify the charge."—*Prof.
Thwing's Facts.*

Miss Laura Bigney, in her prize essay on Tobacco, says :
"The papers recently reported two cases of serious burning
of a young lady and a child, whose clothes had been set on
fire by cigar stubs thrown upon the sidewalk, adding that
the aggravation of the case was only increased by reflecting
that it could not have been the smokers themselves who
were burned."

A single fire in New York, kindled by a smoker's match,
burnt up five blocks and property worth a million dollars !

"One-third, or more, of all the fires in my circuit," says an insurance agent, "have originated from matches and pipes!" Hundreds of similar facts might be given.

"To all this frightful waste must be added the time lost in procuring and using tobacco ; doctors' bills and nurse hire chargeable to the poison ; various apparatus—mouth-pieces, smoking rooms, smoking cars, cigar holders, tobacco boxes, spittoons, pipes, from $\frac{1}{2}$ cent to $1.50 each, etc.; what it costs to dispose of and bring to justice persons led into drunkenness and crime by the use of tobacco ; money paid for extra cleaning necessitated by tobacco filth, and for perfumery to disguise the odor arising therefrom ; the cost which cannot be estimated, but can be only expressed in the terms poverty, stupidity, ignorance, deformity, filth, pain, bodily disease, idiocy, insanity, and death of the bodies and souls of men." Reader, what does the weed cost *you ?*

CHAPTER XIX.

TOBACCO IMPOVERISHES THE SOIL.

" How long shall the land mourn . . . for the wickedness of them that dwell therein ? "—JER. xii. 4.

" THE tobacco plant is a great exhauster. Its organic structure makes it such. Whether raised north or south, on the banks of the Danube or the Connecticut, it is all the same. It is a huge glutton, which, consuming all about it, like Homer's glutton of old, cries ' *more, give me more.*' "

"Tobacco," says Gen. John H. Cooke, of Virginia, "exhausts the land beyond all other crops. As proof of this, every homestead from the Atlantic border to the head of tide-water is a mournful monument. It has been the besom of destruction which has swept over the whole of this once fertile region, producing infinite wretchedness among the people, and turning a fruitful land into barrenness."

A traveller observes: "The old tobacco lands of Maryland and Virginia are an eye-sore, odious 'barrens,' looking as though blasted by some genius of evil."

"An acre of corn and an acre of tobacco are different things to the eye of God or man. Your acre of corn feeds you, your children and your cattle; it creates blood, flesh and bone, and returns in the shape of rich manures, lusty sinews, and grateful hearts, to bless the bosom which nourished it. Your acre of tobacco is chewed and puffed by your fellowmen, who, in defiance of God and Nature, have created a pitiable appetite for it. It makes no blood, no bone, no muscle, and does nothing to nourish the earth, because utterly destitute of the nutritive principle. Such a crop is worthless, because useless. The blast which destroyed the six thousand dollar crop of Col. Colt, in the Connecticut valley, destroyed nothing of intrinsic value. Should God send hail, frost, or fiery foxes through all your tobacco fields and lay all waste, nobody should mourn, for nobody would have lost anything of value."

"Tobacco," says Gen. Cooke, is the bane of Virginia husbandry, because it requires more labor than any other crop, is the most exhausting of all crops, and *is a demoralizer in the broadest sense.*"

" Dr. Humphrey and Dr. Hitchcock, precious men, denounced tobacco raising long ago, and classed it with the business of 'distilling liquid death and damnation.' An eloquent and godly Scotchman moving up and down your

river, ever and anon rebuked this pernicious business in
trumpet tones, in notes of no uncertain sound.   He told you
he had as lief hear the Indian whoop along your valley.   He
had as lief see coffles of slaves delving upon your banks, as
to see your church members, orthodox church members,
professed disciples of Jesus, pursuing a business so completely degrading and destructive!   There are some sins
and crimes which it is not perfectly easy to designate or
name.   You take luxuriant and beautiful soil, which God
designed for the good and happiness of His children, and
desecrate it by a vile crop whose tendency is 'evil and
only evil, and that continually.'   You poison the soil; you
kill the vital principle, and in some sense you murder the
very mother from whose bosom we all draw our nourishment.   Now call this matricide, call it what you please, but
in the light of a better day it will be branded as a sin, a
crime of peculiar magnitude."—*Trask*.

Bishop Huntington, of Central New York, referring to
the culture of tobacco at Hadley, in the Connecticut
valley, a short time ago, states: "Since 1855 enormous
harvests of tobacco have been raised and carried off every
year.   Yet, by the working of some mysterious law, not
one dollar can be found to show for it in all the property
investments or scenery of the entire population."

Another gentleman of large experience, writing on the
same subject, says: "The raising of tobacco has *cursed*
our fair valley.   Hatfield, for instance, some twenty years
ago the richest town in the state according to its population, early entered into the craze for gain through tobacco
raising.   As a result, nearly everyone has failed financially.
But far worse—our farmers, who once declared 'I would
cut off my right hand rather than engage in such a
business,' seeing their neighbors—at the outset—growing

rich, gradually choked conscience and became absorbed in the traffic. This has demoralized the people and paralyzed the church. The spiritual death resting upon this valley may to a great extent be traced to this cause."

Prof. Bascom eloquently writes in reference to what might be expected from its culture. He says: "Take the land, the sunshine, the rain which God gives you, and set them at work to grow tobacco—tobacco that nourishes no man, clothes no man, instructs no man, purifies no man, blesses no man; tobacco that begets inordinate and loathsome appetite and disease and degradation, that impoverishes and debases thousands and adds incalculably to the burden of evil the world bears: but call not this honest trade, or this gnawing at the root of social well-being, getting an honest livelihood. Think of God's justice, the honesty He requires, and cover not your sin with a lie. Turn not His earth and air, given to minister to the sustenance and joy of man, into a narcotic, deadening life and poisoning its current, and then traffic with this for your own good."

CHAPTER XX.

CAN A CHRISTIAN SELL TOBACCO?

"It is good neither to eat flesh, nor to drink wine, nor any thing whereby thy brother stumbleth, or is offended, or is made weak."
—Rom. xiv. 21.

This is an important question. We cannot do better than answer it in the following powerful words of Rev. Geo. Trask :

My Christian Brother,—I answer your inquiry because I presume you wish to know your duty and do it ; and because reform must commence with men like you, who by professions most sacred, are lights of the world. We need your example ; we must have it. The objections to your selling tobacco are very many, and are becoming more and more manifest.

1. *Your Traffic in Tobacco does no good.* This article is neither food, nor drink, nor aliment of any sort ; it does not assimilate with the processes of nature ; it does nothing to build up strength, extend life, or augment the sum total of human happiness. You take money for that which is not bread. You return no equivalent worth the name. Is this kind or honorable? Is this in harmony with the Golden Rule? Are you willing we should take money from your sons for a thing so useless and so vile?

2. *In Selling Tobacco you contribute to a common nuisance.* People of Christian refinement brand the use of it as a filthy practice, polluting earth and air, temples of worship, and the bodies of men—temples of the Holy Ghost. It pollutes your store. Narcotized victims may

not perceive it ; still it is undeniable that this poison permeates your books and bills, your silks and satins, your groceries and every article we buy at your counters. As customers who take pleasure in dealing with you, we ask you, in the name of all that is pure and Christian-like, to drop the sale of it in all forms. It is a nauseous abomination, destined to be driven from all civilized communities as they advance in holiness and towards a millennial state.

3. *The Tobacco you sell Poisons your Customers.* Ask any chemist, any educated physician, and he will tell you that tobacco is a poison—rank and deadly. You may say, "If it be a poison, it is a subtle and insidious one." Be it so ; therefore, it is the more destructive. You may say, "If it be a poison, it is a slow one," It is not so slow but it kills, say physicians, some *twenty thousand* of our countrymen year by year, and strikes down, here and there, its devotees as suddenly as though by a stroke of lightning ! How many sudden deaths around you result from this cause I am unable to state ; but the next neighbor found dead in his field, his office, or his bed, may owe his death to your tobacco ! Boys and men sometimes drop dead, in saloons and stores, whilst chewing and smoking ; and God, my brother, may give you the pain of witnessing such deaths upon your own premises, should you persist in vending this poison ! Deaths by heart-complaints, so called, are rather usually deaths by tobacco !

4. *The Tobacco you sell Creates an Appetite for Strong Drink, Retards the Temperance Reform; and Manufactures Drunkards.*—This point I can with better grace leave you to settle with distinguished physicians.

"A desire is excited," says Dr. Rush, " by tobacco, for strong drinks, and these lead to drunkenness." "Chewing and smoking tobacco," says Dr. Stephenson, "exhaust the

salivary glands, producing dryness and thirst.   Hence,
after the use of a cigar and the quid, brandy, whiskey, or
some other spirit is called for."   Dr. Woodward says, "I
have supposed that tobacco was the common stepping-stone
to that use of spirituous liquors which leads to intemperance."   Hosts of others, whose words should be law,
proclaim the same doctrine.

Be consistent, my brother.   You manifest a noble zeal
against rum-selling ; your store resounds with denunciations
against such traffic.   Why, then, traffic in intoxicating
drugs?   Is it worse to make a man a dolt, an idiot, or
maniac, on one poison than another?   Are not sots sots?
Why manufacture them in any shape?   Why not permit
Satan to do his own work with his own agents?   Why
should a Christian swell the gloomy army of inebriates,
reeling and staggering to perdition ?

5. *In one sense you had better sell Strong Drink than
Tobacco.*—The church and state, heaven and earth, have
been invoked against the one: its evils have been pro-
claimed from the house-tops ; hence he who kills himself
by strong drink, does so against an ocean of light, and
goes down to destruction with his eyes wide open.   But it
is not so with tobacco ; little has been said about it ; its
evils are comparatively unknown ; it is an oily, slimy,
clandestine enemy who does his mischief in silence, and
whose young victims "are caught as fishes in the net, as
birds in the snare."   Secrecy and silence mark the swoop
of this angel of death !

Come, my dear brother, give our children fair play.
Label your poisons by the right name.   Write on your
kegs of snuff, and tobacco, and cigar-boxes, the tendencies
of tobacco.   Write Stupidity ! Laziness ! Poverty ! Vile
Company ! Intemperance ! Crime !   Write Vertigo ! Dyspepsia ! Consumption ! Cancers ! Insanity ! Melancholy !

Delirium Tremens! Sudden Deaths! Suicide! and the loss of the Soul.

Is this severe? Is this extravagant? I assure you the use of tobacco is the great juvenile vice of our times. All forms of incipient iniquity are nursed by its influence. A venerable clergyman calls it "Satan's seed-corn." Significant name! This seed germinates, springs up in diversified forms of blasted hope and melancholy crime! Where is there a vulgar man, where is there a brawny, plunging drunkard, a scape-gallows, not saturated in tobacco!

6. I can name store-keepers who make no pretension to religion, thank God, who have renounced this traffic. They have taken their snuff and cigars, of every hue and odor,—fine-cut, negro-head, and Cavendish, and consigned the whole to the purpose for which God made the poison, —to repel moths and vermin, to kill tick on sheep, and lice on calves. Brother, do the same and God will bless you.

Are you not to be guided, my brother, in this matter, by Christian principle? Does Christ for whom you live sanction this business? Have you sought His guidance? Has He, by word or providence, bid you deal at all in this destructive narcotic?

A young man, on entering business, said to a clergyman, "I believe it is wrong to use strong drink ; is it not wrong to sell it? I believe, also, it is wrong to use tobacco : is it not wrong to sell it? I will sell neither." Noble young man! May God multiply such!

Come, my dear sir, decide at once against this vile branch of merchandise. Men who love Christ, of large and noble views, denounce this traffic more and more. Come, make a clean breast, a clean store ; honor God and gratify customers who abhor this vile weed, and mourn over the evils it inflicts. Be wise. Do not banter nor barter with God, nor with conscience. Yours truly,   G. T.

CHAPTER XXI.

THE DOUBTS OF TOBACCO DEVOTEES.

" Whatsoever is not of faith is sin."—ROM. xiv. 23.

" FOR one inveterate smoker who will bear testimony
favorable to the practice of smoking, ninety-nine are found
to declare their belief that this practice is injurious; and
I scarcely ever yet met with one habitual smoker who did
not, in his candid moments, regret his commencement of
the habit."—*Dr. Johnson.*

Possibly, however, there may be some, who say that they
can smoke and chew with perfect faith in its lawfulness;
and with a conscience clear of any offence. It is clear we
must speak to them in another strain. Let us kindly
inquire of those who claim that they thus use tobacco:
" If you have no doubt now, did your *never* have serious
doubts about this question?" I believe you *have* had such
doubts; and *how* did you settle them? Did you take
them to God? reverently bowing before the Most High for
divine enlightenment? Did you read Romans 14th chap.,
and the 8th, 9th and 10th chap. 1 Cor.? This is the only
way in which Christian men should meet such difficulties.
Did you thus deal with the question, or did you not
endeavor quietly to shelve the whole controversy? Have
you not thus sunk down into a sort of apathetic deadness
of feeling, which is very much like having the conscience
seared? Is it not mere apathy that you mistake for faith
in the propriety of smoking? Let us then ask you to
reconsider the whole question. We candidly confess that

we are anxious to make you *uneasy* in the use of tobacco.
Most earnestly do we beg an answer to the following
queries: Are you *quite sure* that it is right to make use of
a plant or weed which is confessedly one of the rankest
of *poisons?* which, when first used, throws the whole
system into a state of distressing agitation, producing
nausea, headache, prostration of the strength, and a host
of other frightful evils? Are you *satisfied* that it is right
to use what the highest medical testimony, and every-day
experience, tells you tends to sap the vital energies, and
even to enfeeble and ultimately destroy the mental
powers? Are you *positive* that mental science and experience are wrong in this matter, and that your view, on the
contrary, is infallible? Are you *certain* that you are not
robbing God of a part of the strength, physical and mental,
which He claims for himself, by wasting them on a hurtful
indulgence? Are you *quite sure* that your own piety and
spiritual profit have not, in any degree, suffered by your
devotion to this habit? Are you *assured* that you could,
with a clear conscience, teach your wife and children to
smoke? and if you are not, let me ask why? Are you
certain that your usefulness has never suffered, and is not
now suffering, in a single instance, by your love of tobacco?
Are you *satisfied* that this habit of yours has never been a
stumbling stone to a weak brother? Are you *quite sure*
that you have sufficiently weighed the import of this
exhortation: " *Whether, therefore, ye eat or drink, or whatsoever ye do, do all* (smoking and chewing must of course
be included) *to the glory of God.*" (1 Cor. x. 31.) And
remember, that, if you are not *quite sure* with regard to
these queries, you sin in smoking, for " whatsoever is not
of faith is sin."

CHAPTER XXII.

TWELVE PLEAS ANSWERED.

"The hail shall sweep away the refuge of lies," etc.—Isa.
xxviii. 17.

1. "Tobacco cannot be poisonous, as the books allege,
since great numbers who smoke and chew during long life
do not seem to be injured by it."

To this we reply: Many of these objectors, in later
years, have nervous trembling, dyspepsia, heart palpitations, dizziness and sometimes incurable ailments, which
they are astonished to learn from their medical counsel
have been caused chiefly by tobacco. Facts of this sort are
frequent.

It is true, also, that persons of heavy plethoric habits,
and such as live plainly, often perspiring from hard work
in the open air, do not so soon or so severely suffer as
others.

"Suppose that it was well established that men who
kept themselves literally soaked in alcohol had never been
known to have dyspepsia, would it prove that this course
of living was judicious? How could it prevent the difficulty by preserving such a uniform healthy action that
dyspepsia could not appear? Certainly not; but by
creating a so much more powerful morbid condition that
no other disease could well establish itself. There is no
medical man that will deny that tobacco must, in all cases,
whether used as a luxury, or preventive, or cure, create of
itself a morbid action of the system. And it would be
strange policy for the world to adopt, that for fear of some

disease that might come, we must create a disease to forestall it."—*Dr. Coles.*

Some smoke from medicinal motives and to produce a laxative effect, or from absurd notions that it neutralizes neuralgia; but these same persons would grumble loudly at being obliged to take a pill every morning to produce the same effect. If a general order were issued making smoking compulsory, how the fathers of youthful heroes would protest against so very expensive a habit being imposed upon their sons! What an outcry there would be among married ladies for having such an intolerable nuisance forced upon their domestic economy! How the surgeons would be persecuted with applications for certificates recommending exemption from the rule on the score of constitutions being too delicate to admit of smoking being practised with impunity!

It may safely be said that there are other and better preventives of disease than tobacco, and therefore no one is compelled to use the weed for that purpose.

2. "To leave off the use of tobacco would produce a most painful sensation of want."

The appetite has first been formed by yourself. It is not natural, but purely artificial, and that alone should condemn it from a Christian standpoint : it is perfectly needless—not necessary for the sustenance of body or mind.

"When we form bad habits—when we educate the system to love so unnatural an indulgence as the inhalation of the smoke of a deleterious weed, we must expect to suffer for it, both when we begin the process and when we leave it off; nature will have her revenge. If we will behave badly by her, she will punish us for our folly. Very many, in attempting to give up the habit, forget the inconvenience they suffered—how much sleep they lost in forming the habit. They lose sight of the horrid nausea, the nervousness and the host of other evils which they endured in order to become a smoker. They do not reflect on all the inconveniences which they had compelled nature to suffer, against her loud protests, in the process of imitation ; but they conclude that because they had no sleep one night, and seemed unlikely to have any a second night, in attempting to renounce the habit, *ergo*, they could not possibly uneducate the system so as to get it to revert back to its original ability to do without tobacco ! Why should we not be willing to endure as much in breaking off a bad habit as we encountered in forming it? If we punish nature, we must expect nature to punish us. There is this difference, however, between the inconvenience endured in learning to smoke, and that which we have to bear in giving it up—the one resembles the pains which announce the setting up of a disease ; the other is like the pain which sometimes proclaims its departure."

"Some do not give nature a sufficient length of time to return to her normal state, and in this hasty way conclude that the use of tobacco has become a necessity. The very difficulty of the sacrifice only makes its necessity the more apparent, because it demonstrates the positive character of the influence which tobacco has exerted over them. But let all determined smokers remember this, that the greater the difficulty they feel in attempting to renounce the habit, the more urgent the necessity for its abandonment. They must be willing to endure many unpleasant sensations for the first few days. The temporary inconvenience they must boldly face for the sake of the invaluable result to be obtained. They must be resolved to give nature time to recover from the effects of the bad education which she has received at their hands. They have depraved her—they must do their best to rectify her; and if, at first, she be rather rebellious, they must be long-suffering towards her, remembering that they taught her against her will to love the poison."—From *Confessions of an Old Smoker.*

Another mark of an unnatural appetite is, that it secures obedience more by the pain it inflicts when denied, than by the pleasure it confers when indulged.

3. " I take tobacco as a remedy for disease."

Tobacco should not be called a remedy; for there cannot be a doubt that it causes ten thousand diseases where it cures one. Some think they have found relief for phthisical or asthmatic symptoms in tobacco smoke. It is possible that tobacco, by its emetic or narcotic power, may have relieved asthma. But, on the other hand, we have known of asthma being cured by forsaking tobacco, which had been used habitually; and we have the highest medical authority for believing that consumption and bleeding at the lungs have been caused by the habitual use of tobacco. Should it be found, however, that in some extreme case tobacco poison can be used to advantage, is it proper to apply the drug at the mouth?—*Extract.*

Here is what Dr. Coles says on this point : " The use of tobacco by the mouth is in about all cases uncalled for, inexpedient, and even morally wrong. It may sometimes be given by injection, in cases of severe spasmodic diseases with great and beneficial effects. A wet leaf may be introduced into the extremity of the bowel, in case of obstinate colic. It is fit for the fundament, but not for the mouth. Men apply the cigar, the plug, at the wrong extremity of the body. The mouth is no place to stick tobacco."

How long would a man of common sense take the doctor's prescription of any other medicine, and, finding no cure, be willing to continue it ? Would he be willing to take ipecac, calomel or jalap, thirty or forty years, eight or ten doses per day, without any signs of cure ? Tobacco allays the morbid state of stomach, not by creating a healthy action, but by creating a greater morbid action. The tobacco disease is so much greater than the one for which it was taken, that it puts the former complaint into the shade, but does not remove it : it merely covers it up where it is not noticed till the tobacco is discontinued.

1. " The Bible does not say, ' Thou shalt not use tobacco.' " "Because the Bible does not say, 'Thou shalt not feast thyself upon opium, henbane or tobacco,' is it any less a sin to use these articles for such purposes when we learn from the revelation of nature their deadly poison ? A crime against nature is a crime against God. A crime against Divine law, written in nature's book of revelation or rather God's book of nature, in which He reveals His will, may be as fearful in magnitude as a crime against Divine law written in the Bible."

" The Bible is for a different purpose than to teach us facts in science ; and yet all facts in science are as truly of Divine authenticity, and may discover to us Divine obligations as truly as the Bible itself. God's book of nature teaches him who reads it rightly, that tobacco possesses properties of a fearfully deadly character ; that it was not intended as a luxury for man ; that it is contrary to natural instinct ; that it is destroying him and his prosperity and that consequently he ought not to use it. All this is taught as plainly to an intelligent mind, as though it were written in the Holy Volume, " Thou shalt not lust after tobacco."—*Extract.*

" The command is, *Thou shalt love the Lord thy God with all thy heart, with all thy mind, with all thy soul, and with all thy strength*, and I can prove that smoking detracts from physical energy. That which detracts from physical energy must obviously detract from mental energy, and as smoking consumes time and money, smoking prevents compliance with the sacred injunction to love the Lord our God with all our heart, with all our mind, and with all our strength. Thus we have a proof that smoking is a violation of a positive command."—*Thos. Reynolds.*

Such sentences as the following ought to lead to a shrinking from the contact of things which confessedly ruin many of our fellowmen : " Abstain from all appearance of evil." " I keep my body under, and bring it into subjection." " Ye have been called unto liberty, only use not liberty for an occasion to the flesh." " Glorify God in your body and in your spirit which are God's." " If any man defile the temple of God, him shall God destroy." It will be seen, then, that Scripture condemns *all* self-indulgence.

The late Rev. F. H. Robertson well said : " People talk of liberty as if it meant the liberty of doing what a man *likes*. The only liberty a man, worthy the name of a man, ought to ask for, is to have all restrictions, inward and outward, removed, which prevent his doing what he *ought*. I call that man free who is master of his lower appetites, who is able to rule himself. I call him free who has his flesh in subjection to his spirit ; who fears doing wrong, but who fears neither man nor devil besides."

5. " It is so nice to use it." Those who have no better argument than this to use must confess that appetite and not reason leads them. Dr. Mussey relates the following case : " Several years ago, a man applied to me for advice, and commenced a narration of his symptoms, in which I soon interrupted him by saying, ' Sir, you use tobacco,'

'Yes,' he replied, 'I chew a little.' 'Well, sir, do you think it does you any good?' 'No,' said he, 'I think not. I believe on the whole it hurts me.' 'Very well, then, why don't you stop it?' 'Because a man naturally wants a little something, you know, to sweeten his mouth after dinner.' 'Pray, sir, what do you eat for dinner, if that nauseous thing will sweeten your mouth?'"

The great difficulty with all sinners is, that they are governed by appetite and not by reason—they are led by the law of sin in their members, rather than by conscience and the blessed will of God—"Walking after their own lusts."

How can persons who use such a plea as this profess to be "walking after the Spirit," to "have crucified the flesh with the affections and lusts?" Does not the apostle emphatically state that "if ye live after the flesh ye shall die?"

6. "How comes it that so many years have elapsed since Sir Walter Raleigh first made smoking fashionable, and yet the practice has not wrought the evil deprecated, to the amount which might have been expected!"

Although centuries have elapsed since the introduction of tobacco into Europe, invention so rife in the present day, has given in our time a mighty impetus to this baneful habit. Until within the last few years tobacco was usually consumed through a long clay pipe, which was subjected to frequent purifications by fire. The comparatively recent introduction of fancy pipes and cigars, while it has facilitated the use of the article in question, has also augmented its deleterious effects.

The fancy pipe favors the accumulation of oil in the act of smoking, causing the diversion to be more intensely detrimental to health than when pursued by the long clay pipes of our grandfathers' days.

Another simple invention has also conduced to the popularity of the habit. A tinder-box, flint and steel, and a bundle of sulphur-tipped slips of wood, would be cumbrous appliances to participating in the luxury, and being compelled to employ such in conjunction with the long pipe, would deter many a little lad from the imitative joy; he "would shrink from the world's dread laugh, which not even the stern philosopher could bear."

Again, our stern grandsires put off tobacco smoking till after the substantial English dinner, which would neutralize in a measure the acrid poison.

The boys, to whom the habit is especially detrimental, had not begun the puffing sin; hence, judgment upon the obnoxious effects of tobacco smoking must be suspended for at least a generation.

7. "It would be prejudicial to health to renounce the habit."

Says Dr. Lizars: "A remarkable change occurs to the smoker when he labors under influenza or fever, as he then not only loses all relish for the pipe, but actually loathes it.

"The sudden removal of all desire to smoke, affords the best refutation to the delusive representation which the unhappy victim of tobacco urges for continuing the injurious habit, on the ground that its abandonment would be prejudicial to his health, and proves that if he had a will to relinquish the pipe or cigar, he could find a way.

"The best argument to use in dealing with the obstinate prejudices of such people is to tell them that an accidental attack of a new disease can safely and at once occasion the total withdrawal of tobacco without producing any bad consequences.

"It is scarcely possible to cure either syphilis or gonorrhœa if the patient continues to indulge in tobacco."

Says another physician : "The chewing of tobacco is not necessary or useful in any case that I know of, and I have abundant evidence that its use may be discontinued without pernicious consequences."

Dr. Laycock, Professor of the Practice of Physics in the University of Edinburgh, has this to say : "I have not known any good from tobacco that might not have been obtained from less objectionable means."

8. "The doctor ordered me to smoke."

Yes, but that is to patients. We never heard of it curing anyone—not very effective medicine to be taken for life.

Did those who were ordered to smoke give up the weed when their allotted time for its use expires, it would be different ; but what are the facts ?

In the majority of instances those who receive such instructions continue to indulge in the weed after the prescribed period for its use as a medicine has expired ; and under cover of the physician's order, still infuse the poison into their systems. Some of the very best of the medical profession have never been known to order the use of tobacco. For one *bona fide* case of doctor-ordering, are there not hundreds of shams ?

Experience shows that the doctor is often compelled to give in to the whim of a weak or refractory patient.

9. "I cannot hear to advantage without tobacco ; it quickens my attention, and I profit more by the sermon." Dr. Adam Clarke says : "I am disposed to think there is some truth in this, and such persons exactly resemble those who have habituated themselves to frequent doses of opium,

who, from the well-known effect of a free use of the drug, are in a continual torpor except for a short time after each dose. Thus they are obliged to have constant recourse to a stimulant which in proportion to its use increases the disease. Such persons as these are unfit to appear in the house of God! This conduct proves that they are wholly destitute of the spirit of piety and of a sense of their spiritual wants, when they need such excitement to help their devotions."

10. "Why did God send tobacco?" This question is more curious than profitable; nor is it, we fear, the outcome of a candid spirit anxious to know the right thing and do it. As well might we ask, why did God make the wasp, the viper, the crocodile, the shark? Had we that infinite knowledge possessed by the Creator, we should see that He made everything "beautiful in its season." What if in certain plants reside latent properties which man can pervert to the injury of himself or his neighbor, is God therefore unwise, unrighteous? Does He instruct His creature man to use these properties for evil? Is man perforce constrained to take Virginia's fair green plant, to twist to "pigtail," to torture and torment to "negro-head," to cut and shred into "returns" and "shag," compress and roll into cigars, and pulverize into snuff, and use it as Satan's agent to work woe and sin? Right well we know that there are many things in creation which can be turned to man's advantage; but he who, from the fact of finding the plant in nature, would therefore assume that he had a sanction to kill it, in order to manufacture and produce a poisonous drug, wherewith to afflict his fellowmen, and fill his own coffers, would be acting as wisely as he who should fire a house or stack, thereby spreading destruction and misery around, and as the justification for

9

his crime should sagely relate how in early childhood he had seen his aged grandmother evoke from antiquated flint and steel a spark of fire, which falling upon the tindered material had become the means of lighting the fire with which to prepare the morning meal.

But is everything that is made, or in other words, every-thing that is a natural product, everything that grows on the soil, to be used as a luxury? If so, opium grows, and therefore should be chewed, or otherwise habitually used.

Deadly nightshade and henbane are productions of nature; and should these, therefore, become habitual luxuries?

11. "Great and good men smoke and chew." Yes, some of the great and good of our land do use the weed, but what does this prove—that it is right to use tobacco? Certainly not. The best of men err, and sometimes grievously, too. The example of the holiest of men is not to be copied further than those examples agree with the Word of God. We have seen that the common use of tobacco is condemned by the Bible, therefore the example of no tobacco devotee, however deep his piety (?) should be followed. It is at least very questionable whether a single *good* man can be found—be he a consumer of tobacco or not—who could cheerfully and sincerely recommend the use of the weed.

Persons who for a great many years have been addicted to the weed, in their dying moments give emphatic testi-mony against the use of the drug. Says a minister: "I called on a dying man, a member of my church. He said that tobacco had brought him to his death-bed, and he should die a happier man if he left his testimony in writing against this sin. I wrote from his dictation, and he gave it his signature. My reflections were painful. A dying brother giving his testimony against a sin of which I, his pastor, am guilty ! Oh, then, I called God to witness that I renounced tobacco for ever ! "

Last, but not least, the example of Christ is against the habit. Who can imagine for one moment our blessed Lord and Master (whose example we are to imitate) going about with a dirty, stinking tobacco pipe in His mouth, and while consoling words proceed from His sacred lips to disconsolate souls, the fumes of tobacco smoke proceeding therefrom ?

12. "Tea is as bad as tobacco." We believe the use of tea to be very injurious to the nervous system, but it is not to be compared with tobacco. If you doubt this the following experiment would soon convince you : Put in your tea-pot the same quantity of tobacco and water which you would in preparing tea. Take a cupful of it with milk and sugar. If it did not kill you it would make you helplessly drunk.

" If any parallel exists between theine in tea, and the principles in tobacco, there can be no parallel in its *effect*. Theine in tea is, as ordinarily employed, diluted to the extent of some hundreds per cent. Tobacco undergoes *no such dilution :* therefore, there is as much differance between theine in tea, and tobacco fumes, as exists between fire and water."

CHAPTER XXIII.

PROGRESS OF THE ANTI-TOBACCO MOVEMENT.

THE late Rev. Geo. Trask, of Fitchburg, Mass., devoted some twenty-five years of his active life mainly to warring against the widely spread, and ever growing tobacco nuisance.

Anti-tobacco societies have recently been formed in France, England, Russia, Montreal and some in the United States. Most of these societies are gaining ground. Some anti-tobacco book and tract societies have of late been opened on this continent. The Board of Public Instruction in Paris has issued a circular forbidding the use of tobacco by students in the public schools of that city. In Germany the police in several states have been instructed to stop all smoking by lads and young men. This action is based on the testimony of the medical faculty that tobacco using is so injurious to the health as to impair the fitness of boys and young men for the military service, in which, in Germany, all young men must bear a part.

The progress of smoking in South Australia has been so great within recent years that it has been thought advisable to attempt to check its growth among the youth. A measure has therefore been introduced into the House of Assembly to the effect that any person under the age of eighteen who shall smoke any pipe, cigar or cigarette shall be guilty of an offence, and, on conviction, shall be liable to a penalty of not less than 5s., nor more than £5; and in default of payment, may be imprisoned for any time not exceeding one month. Whenever any person shall be charged, the onus of proving the age shall, in all cases, lie on the person so charged. One-half of every penalty imposed is to be paid to the informer, the remainder to the treasurer for the public use of the province.

The Senate of New Jersey has recently imposed a fine of twenty dollars on any person convicted of selling tobacco to minors; this because of the prevalence of smoking among small boys.

Vermont and several other states, also Switzerland, have also commenced to legislate against tobacco.

At the West Point Military School, U.S., the Superintendent, General O. Howard, has forbidden the use of tobacco by the cadets.

In England the use of tobacco has been prohibited within the precincts of Windsor Castle by the express command of Her Majesty the Queen. Many leading English newspapers, and other prominent publications, are now frequently denouncing the common use of this poison. Eminent physicians all over Europe and America are raising their united testimony against the vile weed. Bishops, ministers of all denominations, lawyers, school teachers, and others in public positions, are making earnest efforts in their respective spheres to baffle this giant foe. Railway companies, not a few, are prosecuting offenders for smoking in non-smoking carriages, heavy fines being inflicted in nearly every case. Coal-miners are also taught that smoking in their pits cannot be allowed—some having been imprisoned for so doing. Several cases of this kind have recently been reported by the English papers. School teachers are finding out that non-smoking pupils succeed best. A wedding in Rome, N.Y., was indefinitely postponed because the young man in the case declined to give up the use of tobacco.

In Seville, O., the young ladies formed an anti-tobacco society. They have pledged themselves to have nothing to do with any young gentleman so lost to decency as to use the vile drug! Other signs of progress have developed more fully of late:

1. Many ecclesiastical bodies have discussed the *morality* of using tobacco, and taken action upon it as *immoral* and *sinful*. Nearly every section of the Christian church has recently voted against their ministers using the weed. In the admittance of members they act accordingly—not allowing anyone to be a member that uses the weed. Even the Mormons have a rule against it. Many parishes have decided to discharge youthful aspirants to the pulpit the devotees of smoke—wishing less smoke and more fire. A gentleman in Russia, of high rank, some time ago informed us that 13,000,000 of Orthodox Dissenters in Russia believe that smoking tobacco is a sin.

2. Rich men, in legacies to colleges and schools, begin to restrict their benefactions to students who have nothing to do with this and similar vices—not wishing that their money should evaporate in smoke.

3. Merchants in advertising for clerks, announce that smokers and striplings of this stripe "need not apply;" "Havanas" are costly.

4. Store-keepers, who *have consciences*, begin to think it *dishonorable* to sell this nuisance, and to take money from ragged youths and paupers for "that which is not bread."

5. Bands of hope, pledged against strong drink, tobacco and profaneness, are rapidly spreading. A flourishing band of hope has recently been organized in Calcutta, India, whose pledge is against tobacco and strong drink.

In many temperance organizations vigorous efforts are now being made against this great ally of old Alcohol.

6. The legislature of Ontario has recently enacted a law forbidding the sale of tobacco to children under eighteen years of age under a penalty of not less than ten dollars or more than fifty dollars, or imprisonment for thirty days.

7. One of the most encouraging signs of the progress of the anti-narcotic crusade in the United States is the establishment of a " National Anti-Narcotic Department " by the Woman's Christian Temperance Union.

8. The discipline of the Free Methodist Church of Canada and of the United States forbids any of its members to use, grow, or manufacture tobacco. This rule is rigidly enforced.

9. It has been recently suggested that railway directors have smoking cars labelled, **"FOR THE UNCLEAN,"** and allow none but smokers and chewers to enter them.

10. Missionary tidings from distant lands inform us that those who would win the heathen from their darkness to Christ *must* have *clean* hands and *pure* hearts. One report reads : " For God's sake, keep your *wretched stuff* at home and don't degrade my people."♦ Another states : " If the *cursed weed* and *fire water* you bring to us are the fruits of Christianity, we don't want it." Even the benighted Hindoo brands Christians in his land who use tobacco or spirits as "drunkards " to be shunned.

11. At the recent yearly meeting of the Society of Friends, held at Raleigh, North Carolina, 1894, the following report of the temperance committee was adopted : " We recommend that in the future no member of the Society of Friends of North Carolina shall be recorded as a minister, or appointed an elder, who engages in the use of tobacco."

12. Rev. Joseph Cook says: "There was recently an examination for candidates for admission to a church in Japan, and a prominent preacher there, Mr. Tse, put to a candidate for admission the question whether he used tobacco. The reply being in the affirmative, the preacher said, 'All purity becomes a Christian. I shall advise you not to unite with the church until you give up tobacco.' The convert gave up the weed."

That this movement is, under God, steadily advancing, we infer from the fact that considerable opposition has been aroused by the circulation of our anti-tobacco publications. Ministers, editors, and hundreds of smoking and chewing professors have written and said strong things against us and our work. Abuse, scorn and slander have been heaped upon us, and diligent efforts made to frustrate our labors.

In November, 1882, we received an anonymous letter from some person who, it seems, had been presented through the mail with a variety of tracts, including some of our own, on Masonry, Tobacco, Popery, and other popular sins. These tracts so stirred up his wrath, that he returned two of them to us and wrote us a letter, which, for bitter, foul language, falsehoods, and insinuations of gross immorality, we have seldom seen equalled. From the language of his letter, it is evident he must have been boiling with rage. But, instead of feeling any resentment towards him, we deeply pitied the poor slave to sin, and rejoiced that we were counted worthy to suffer reproach and slander for Christ's sake. We did, indeed, find that "*Blessed* are they which are persecuted for righteousness' sake, "etc., for we were made wonderfully happy in God, and went from the post office singing and praising the Lord. We frequently hear the devotees of these popular idols plead that there is no harm in them; yea, they would have us believe they are even scriptural; but look! just as soon as one gives a little light on these things, they are full of indignation and revenge. They thus give the plainest proof of their guilt; for, if their practices were as good and pure as they would have the public believe, they would not hate the light and be so enraged when they are exposed. But, says the Bible: "Men love darkness rather than light *because their deeds are evil.*"

However, as God has been pleased to give us His blessing and to crown our efforts with success, we are devoutly thankful; and in the name of God will push this battle on. We must, we will, scatter the truth, and reach precious souls if we can.

CHAPTER XXIV.

FIFTY-FOUR OBJECTIONS TO TOBACCO.

1. Tobacco was one main upholder of Slavery in the United States of America.
2. Tobacco and its appendages cost the United Kingdom at least £11,000,000 a year.
3. Tobacco when first smoked, chewed or snuffed, offends the whole system.
4. Tobacco contains an essential oil and nicotine, both of which are highly poisonous.
5. Tobacco exerts a special influence on the brain and the nervous system generally.
6. Tobacco seriously affects the action of the heart and circulation of the blood.

7. Tobacco, by perverting the nourishing saliva, prevents due elaboration of chyle and blood.

8. Tobacco, by weakening the nerves, produces morbid excitability and irritability.

9. Tobacco impairs the senses of smelling and tasting, and often of hearing and seeing.

10. Tobacco when freely used, depresses the energies of the mind, and leads to despondency.

11. Tobacco arrests the growth of the young, and thereby lowers the stature.

12. Tobacco when smoked by boys, causes a craving for it, to gratify which they lie or steal.

13. Tobacco in numerous instances weakens the memory, and thereby tends to insanity.

14. Tobacco, by undermining physical vigor, causes the keepers of the house to tremble.

15. Tobacco has a tendency to loosen the silver cord, and superinduces paralysis.

16. Tobacco harms the gums and teeth, and the grinders cease because they are few.

17. Tobacco weakens every function and fibre of the human frame by poisoning the blood.

18. Tobacco is a known cause of enfeeblement to the posterity of its consumers.

19. Tobacco is an acknowledged cause of demoralization to the young of all classes.

20. Tobacco smoked, chewed or snuffed, deceives by causing delusive imaginations.

21. Tobacco hastens the evil day in which many say, "I have no pleasure in them."

22. Tobacco is expensive, and if wives and children want food, the pipe must be filled.

23. Tobacco smoking occasions great waste of time, "The stuff which life is made of."

24. Tobacco keeps many of its besotted victims in a state of habitual semi-intoxication.

25. Tobacco is a great promoter of drinking customs, by creating unnatural thirst.

26. Tobacco, by its exhausting and depressing power, renders strong drink a necessity.

27. Tobacco is the admitted cause of multitudes breaking the Total Abstinence pledge.

28. Tobacco is therefore a great hindrance to the progress of Temperance Reform.

29. Tobacco smoking is the only vice uncondemned from the Pulpit, Press and Platform.

30. Tobacco doubtless causes many fires which come under the head of "Cause Unknown."

31. Tobacco pollutes the breath, and unfits its consumers for refined society.

32. Tobacco is a class breaker, and greatly tends to lead its victims into bad associations.

33. Tobacco frequently induces habits of indolence, apathy and listless inactivity.

34. Tobacco consumers are more liable to disease than if they were in a natural condition.

35. Tobacco weakens the constitution, and renders recovery from sickness a great difficulty.

36. Tobacco, by weakening mental perception, leaves its victims an easy prey to tempters.

37. Tobacco being much in demand, induces many to keep their shops open on Sunday.

38. Tobacco mars beauty, destroys the complexion, and impairs the brilliancy of the eyes.

39. Tobacco smoked, chewed or snuffed, is opposed to the politeness of a gentleman.

40. Tobacco, as James the First said, bewitches him that useth it. He cannot leave it off.

41. Tobacco, by *enfeebling* the *will*, becomes a *prolific* cause of *irresolution*.

42. Tobacco is at variance with the dictates which Christianity inspires in the soul.

43. Tobacco robs the pulpit by circumscribing the qualifications of smoking ministers.

44. Tobacco robs the pew and Sunday School of multitudes who smoke that day away.

45. Tobacco begets strife in railway carriages, ale and temperance houses, and home circles.

46. Tobacco, by robbing workingmen, clothes many of them and their children with rags.

47. Tobacco smoked in confined rooms, is very injurious to sickly women and children.

48. Tobacco is very powerful in leading to forgetfulness of God and the duty of self-denial.

49. Tobacco has caused many parents to exclaim, "Would God I had died for thee, my son."

50. Tobacco has done much to fill poor-houses, hospitals and lunatic asylums.

51. Tobacco and drinks which its use demands, cost enough to evangelize the world.

52. Tobacco and drinks are causes of long credit for articles of necessity and utility.

53. Tobacco greatly detracts from the honor of God, by frustrating His benevolent designs.

54. Finally, to young and old we say, Touch Not Tobacco, for a Curse is in it.

CHAPTER XXV.

CHRISTIAN LADIES *VS.* TOBACCO.

THE following powerful appeal to Christian ladies was written by Rev. George Trask. We fervently hope every lady will ponder well these weighty words :

" We asked a Christian lady to contribute a little money to spread tracts over the nation, and save our youth from being destroyed by tobacco. She broke into smiles of provoking indifference, exclaiming : 'Why, my husband smokes, my sons smoke! It is a filthy habit ; but it makes them easy and happy, and if they do nothing worse, they may smoke to their hearts' content!' Our churches abound with ladies in this or similar states of mind ; and such I now address.

"Ladies, tobacco is a deceptive demon. Like other demons, he has his peculiar 'wiles,' and his 'depths you have not known.' We shall not spread this evil before you in its manifold bearings, but only call your attention to three questions, which we beg you duly to consider.

" 1. *Ladies, do you know that the attachment of your friends to tobacco is absolutely idolatrous? That they probably love it better than they love you?* If they use much, and have used it long, this is a fair inference. And you here have a rival which is more than a match for you. This appetite is artificial, created in defiance of every law and instinct of nature ; hence it is a monstrosity, in point of strength, and easily binds its victims in chains invincible.

" The drunkard prefers his pipe to his bottle ; the glutton prefers his tobacco with one meal a day to three without it. The politician, disappointed at the polls, finds consolation in his cigar, not in his wife. Ladies, you ring the changes on the filthiness of this thing, but your friends prefer it to the finest delicacies you spread before them, or to the whole magnificent array of luxuries which God pours around them from every clime. Money, strong drink and opium have no such charms. The love of it sometimes rises to the dignity of a passion, swaying its victim hither and thither in life, and showing itself to be the ruling passion strong in death ! We maintain that the love of it exceeds 'the love of woman.' Many use it when they know and confess they are committing suicide ; hence, they love it better than life. But do they love you, ladies, better than life ? Rob your husband of this idol forty-eight hours and he becomes peevish and porcupinish, and it is well if he does not make a Bedlam of your house ! A merchant in a city near by us, deprived of his tobacco a day or two, became infuriated to madness, and inflicted kicks on his wife and children without mercy ! No rare case. Mothers, your sons love you, but they love their idols better. Your husband, should he follow you to the grave, would weep and mourn ; but, if he is like other tobacco sots he could forget you more easily than his tobacco. Among the possibilities, he might find a substitute for you ; but in the name of all the sons of smoke up and down the globe, we ask, where, Oh ! where is there a substitute for tobacco ? There is many a fine girl who, should she say to her lover, 'Give up tobacco totally and for ever, or give up me,' would soon learn that she has a rival who has the throne and will keep it !

" Ladies, we have no wish to move you to jealousy ; but you profess to be Christian women, and when we see you treat anti-tobacco efforts with scornful indifference, we are compelled to ask, are you willing that 'lover and friend' should use tobacco 'to their hearts' content,' when they bestow upon it more time, more attention, love and admiration than they bestow upon you?

"2. *Ladies, do you know that tobacco in your families may poison you, your children, and your posterity?* Men of sense say but little about it as a nuisance. They go deeper; they treat it as a rank poison, which penetrates flesh and blood and bone, becoming part and parcel of the man, making him a living receptacle of the virus, a poisoned body, which, whether asleep or awake, at home or abroad, by insensible perspiration, poisons the common air we breathe. The tobacco effluvia of your son is sufficient to make a stage-load of women and children sick who are not accustomed to it. The tobacco your husband uses each day, made into tea and given to a score of children, would poison the whole, and probably lay many of them dead! The effects of a bit the size of a bean, found in a tea-pot, once alarmed a whole village! It had poisoned the tea, and the tea had poisoned a whole maternal association! These precious ladies found 'death in the pot,' and they began to suspect tobacco had killed them, whether it had or had not killed their husbands. Take the water from the tub in which a tobacco devotee has been steaming, apply it to the geraniums over town, and it will soon despatch the vermin, and geraniums, too, unless applied with care!

"Ladies, we are not attempting to show that the users of tobacco injure themselves; this would be superfluous; but do they injure others? Do they injure you and your children? We think they do. Fathers beget children in their own likeness. They transmit their color, features, forms, temperaments and diseases, and sometimes their appetites. And the idea that the offspring of parents debauched on rum, or debauched on tobacco, can avoid the disabilities of birth, or avoid an internal law of God, is ridiculous, is pitiable. Physicians of acumen and sense have sometimes pointed us to family after family of dwarfs and half idiots, saying in substance, 'These are specimens of the inherited effects of tobacco! The parents were sots on the poison; like begets like, and here you have it!' Physicians and others have now and then named the case of an infant here and there, which actually inherited a taste for tobacco, and their wailings, when a few days old, were actually appeased by beastly parents actually applying tobacco to their tongues! A splendid woman remarks, 'If getting married does not reform the tobacco toper, one of its blessed effects ought to do so, for no man ought to poison his babe!'

"Mothers, you have lost young children; they grew sick and died strangely, and no satisfactory cause was assigned which robbed you of these objects of endearment. But did it ever occur to you, that, as soon as born, your babes were enveloped in tobacco smoke, and their tender lungs played in a poisoned atmosphere the instant they began to play at all? Did it ever occur to you that your child, by sleeping with its father, slept with a huge body of poison, perspiring at a million pores, and lodging in exhalations on the babe? Alas! alas! many fathers of tearful eyes and noble hearts have killed their own children without knowing it!

"Mothers! Rachels! you who have rebelled against God, you who have filled the air with wailings for children which are no more—children killed by the very one who loves them most, the father—are you willing that husbands and sons 'should smoke to their hearts' content if they do nothing worse'?

" 3. *Ladies, do you know that tobacco tends to hinder salvation, and to destroy the souls of those you love?* To devote the soul to God, and accept Christ in a saving manner, mind should be awake, rational, and no way disturbed and confused by drugs or drinks. A college of physicians testify to the disturbing power of tobacco. 'Tobacco,' they say, 'abnormalizes and hallucinates mind. A hard drinker may soon arise from his debauch, and be himself again ; but not so with the habitual user of tobacco, for he is always under its effects, and hence always in an abnormal state !'

" Tobacco, used in some forms, excites and exasperates, in others stupefies and stultifies. When smoked it tends to deaden sensibility and fill the soul with self-satisfaction. The smoker, whilst sublimely fumigating earth and air, is satisfied ! He is satisfied, whether rich or poor, married or single—he has a pipe ! He is satisfied whether in the forecastle or cabin, whether at the head of a factory or an understrapper—he has a pipe ! He is satisfied whether he knows much or little, whether saint or sinner—he has a pipe !

" Ladies, such is the power of this narcotic, that you perceive its effects on religion must be very disastrous. Look over the churches and you will see mournful specimens of its effects. See for yourselves. On the one hand there is a brother who is actually better known as a smoker than a Christian. He is proverbially clever. He makes no difficulties. He likes the minister ; he likes the deacons, and is proud of the architecture of the church. He is always comfortably seated in his pew ; and whether the discourse be from Calvary or Sinai, it is all the same, he enjoys it, providing he has previously enjoyed his pipe, for his piety takes the type of his pipe. Now, ladies, this cipher in the church, this stupefied man that does nothing for God or

10

his race, is your brother; you sprung from the same parents! Are you willing he should 'smoke to his heart's content, if he does nothing worse'? There is a church-member, lank and lean, who professes to eschew evil, but who chews tobacco with a vengeance. He is nervous, irritable, and misanthropic, and abounds with what Wesley calls 'Satan's religion—a sour religion.' In his view, everything is 'all out of sorts'—minister, deacons, taxes, and all, and he has no comfort in his life. What is the matter with the brother? He chews. Who is he? He is your husband! Are you willing that he should chew tobacco 'if he does nothing worse'?

"There is a young man, who has abandoned your Bible-class, and well-nigh abandoned the house of God; but he is not a drunkard, nor blasphemer, nor gambler, nor heretic. He, however, smokes and chews, and Saturday evening he procures a double stock, and on Sabbath he smokes, sleeps and lounges about, satisfied to let other people carry on divine worship, providing he is well supplied with 'fine cut,' and cigars! Dear, respected mother, this young man is your son, and are you willing that he should chew and smoke 'if he does nothing worse'?

"Ladies, look a little higher. There stands a preacher, a man of talents and culture. He has capacities to do an aggressive work and make all things new around him. But he fails as a pastor, because he wishes to be ensconced in his study, to smoke! He does not exchange much, because he cannot smoke abroad as he smokes at home! He does not mingle in reforms, because his easy-chair, his cigars and his polite literature have superior charms! He attends a few funerals and weddings, he preaches a few sermons; and, though he ought to live and toil for Christ till threescore and ten, he dies at forty and is seen no more!

This, ladies, may be your own preacher ! We have thousands of such ! Are you willing that your pastor and the bishop of your souls should 'chew and smoke to his heart's content, if he does nothing worse' ?

"An eminent physician of Boston thus addresses you : 'Ladies, you have the highest interest in this question, one involving the health and the lives of yourselves and families. Permit me to say that you have the power to do what gentlemen are unable to do. You can banish this curse from the community. Ponder, Resolve, and Act.'

"Act, ladies, act ! 1. Denounce the use of tobacco as a sin. 2. Spread tracts against it. 3. Remonstrate against raising it or selling it. 4. Do as others have done, object to settling a minister who is a slave to it. 5. Object to your daughters marrying slaves to it.

"It is with us a matter of joy and pride that our wives and daughters are not the victims of tobacco, that they all, who honor womanhood, move queenlike above this vile pollution, this vile servitude. Thank God, we have this line of demarkation, well defined and visible between noble women and sensual men !

"We gladly acknowledge the aid we have in our work, from here and there a mother in Israel—or a Christian and patriotic woman. They pray--they work - they give.

"We have women who battle with pernicious habits 'might and main,' often with marked success. We have women who see as clearly as we see, that there is no hope of our young men reaching Christ, or the members of our churches reaching heaven, whilst slaves to this lust.

"They begin to see that the Gospel cannot take effect where moral agency is paralyzed by opium and tobacco. And so long as vast nations like China and Turkey are crushed to earth by the stupefying and stultifying power of such baleful drugs, they cannot rise to God, and the conversion of the world must remain a hopeless undertaking.

"We trust the time is at hand when both the sons and daughters of Zion throughout the Church will see that opium and tobacco are mighty obstructions to the advancing kingdom, and do something worth the name for their removal."

CHAPTER XXVI.

MISCELLANEOUS FACTS.

Tobacco—A Parable.—Then shall the kingdom of Satan be likened to a grain of tobacco seed, which, though exceeding small, being cast into the ground grew, and became a great plant, and spread its leaves rank and broad, so that huge and vile worms formed a habitation thereon. And it came to pass, in the course of time, that the sons of men looked upon it, and thought it beautiful to look upon, and much to be desired to make lads look big and manly. So they did put forth their hands and did chew thereof. And some it made sick, and others to vomit most filthily. And it further came to pass that those who chewed it became weak and unmanly, and said we are enslaved and can't cease from chewing it. And the mouths of all that were enslaved became foul and they were seized with a violent spitting; and they did spit, even in ladies' parlors, and in the house of the Lord of hosts. And the saints of the Most High were greatly plagued thereby. And in the course of time it came also to pass that others snuffed it;

and they were taken suddenly with fits, and they did sneeze
with a great and mighty sneeze, insomuch that their eyes
filled with tears, and they did look exceedingly silly. And
yet others cunningly wrought the leaves thereof into rolls,
and did set fire to the one end thereof, and did suck
vehemently at the other end thereof, and did look very
grave and calf-like; and the smoke of their torment
ascended up forever and ever.

And the cultivation thereof became a great and mighty
business on the earth : and the merchantmen waxed rich
by the commerce thereof. And it came to pass that the
saints of the Most High defiled themselves therewith : even
the poor who could not buy shoes, nor bread, nor books for
their little ones, spent their money for it. And the Lord
was greatly displeased therewith and said : "Wherefore
this waste : why do these little ones lack bread, and shoes
and books? Turn now your fields into corn and wheat,
and put this evil thing far from you ; and be separate, and
defile not yourselves any more : and I will bless you and
cause my face to shine on you."

But with one accord they all exclaimed : "We cannot
cease from chewing, snuffing and puffing—we are slaves."
—*Christian Secretary.*

The representative of a large tobacco house in the South,
says that the extent to which drugs are used in "doctor-
ing" cigarettes is appalling.

"The drugs impart a sweet and pleasant flavor and have
a soothing effect, that in a little time obtain a fascinating
control over the smoker. The more cigarettes he smokes
the more he desires to smoke, as is the case with one who
uses opium. The desire grows to a passion. The smoker
becomes a slave to the enervating habit. To the insidious
effects of the drugs is attributed the success of the cigarette.

"By the use of drugs it is possible to make a very inferior quality of tobacco pleasant. Manufacturers, therefore, put these vile things on the market at a price that makes it easy for the poorest to indulge in their killing delights, and boys and youths go in swarms for them.

"What is called 'Havana Flavoring' has grown to be an important article of commerce. Thousands of barrels of it are sold everywhere. It is extensively used in manufacturing certain kinds of cigarettes. It is made from the tonca bean, which contains a drug called mellolotis, a deadly poison, seven grains of which will kill a dog. Imagine the effect which must result from puffing that vile stuff into the lungs hour after hour.

"The paper coverings manufactured from filthy scrapings of rag-pickers are also a fruitful source of evil to the cigarette smoker. Vile as it is, it is bought up in great masses by agents of the manufacturers, who turn it into the dingy pulp and subject it to a bleaching process to make it presentable. The lime and other substances used in bleaching have a very harmful influence upon the membrane of the mouth, throat and nose, and it is so cheap that a thousand cigarettes can be wrapped with it at a cost of two cents.

"Arsenical preparations, it is said, are used in bleaching most cigarette papers, and oil of creosote is produced naturally as a consequence of combustion. The latter has a most injurious effect upon the membrane of the mouth, throat and lungs, and it is said to accelerate the development of consumption in anyone predisposed to the disease.

"A mouthpiece which had been in use was unrolled by a smoker. Its edge, to the depth of about half an inch, was covered with the dark, poisonous acid, the odor of which was intolerable. The pernicious stuff, taken into smokers' systems, assists to bring about the sunken cheeks, the dull and listless appearance which mark the slave of the cigarette."—*Philadelphia Times.*

The following dissipation interest table is, by permission, taken from an interesting pamphlet by Chester E. Pond, entitled "*A Tornado Among the Human Tobacco Shrubs.*" A careful perusal will show the reader the immense waste caused by the indulgence in tobacco.

Suppose your average dissipation amounts to only five cents a day for tobacco, then during the

First Year you wasted........................	$18 25
Second Year you lose Interest Money	1 09 5
And, at **Five Cents per day**, you waste	18 25
In Two years you have wasted and lost	$37 59 5
Third Year you lose Interest Money	2 25 5
And, at **Five Cents per day**, you waste	18 25
In Three years you have wasted and lost......	$58 10
Fourth Year you lose Interest Money...........	3 48 6
And, at **Five Cents per day**, you waste	18 25
In Four years you have wasted and lost	$79 83 6
Fifth Year you lose Interest Money	4 79
And, at **Five Cents per day**, you waste	18 25
In Five years you have wasted and lost	$102 87 6
Sixth Year you lose Interest Money	6 17 2
And, at **Five Cents per day**, you waste	18 25
In Six years you have wasted and lost	$127 29 8
Seventh Year you lose Interest Money	7 63 7
And, at **Five Cents per day**, you waste.......	18 25
In Seven years you have wasted and lost	$153 18 5
Eighth Year you lose Interest Money...........	9 19 1
And, at **Five Cents per day**, you waste.......	18 25
In Eight years you have wasted and lost	$180 62 6
Ninth Year you lose Interest Money	10 83 7
And, at **Five Cents per day**, you waste	18 25
In Nine years you have wasted and lost	$209 71 3
Carried forward,	$209 71 3

☞ The figures at the right indicate mills, or tenths of a cent.

Amount brought forward,	\$209	71	3
Tenth Year you lose Interest Money	12	58	2
And, at **Five Cents per day,** you waste.......	18	25	
In Ten years you have wasted and lost........	\$240	54	5
Eleventh Year you lose Interest Money..........	14	43	2
And, at **Five Cents per day,** you waste	18	25	
In Eleven years you have wasted and lost	\$273	22	7
Twelfth Year you lose Interest Money	16	39	3
And, at **Five Cents per day,** you waste......	18	25	
In Twelve years you have wasted and lost	\$307	87	
Thirteenth Year you lose Interest Money	18	47	2
And, at **Five Cents per day,** you waste	18	25	
In Thirteen years you have wasted and lost....	\$344	59	2
Fourteenth Year you lose Interest Money........	20	67	5
And, at **Five Cents per day,** you waste.......	18	25	
In Fourteen years you have wasted and lost....	\$383	51	7
Fifteenth Year you lose Interest Money..........	23	01	1
And, at **Five Cents per day,** you waste	18	25	
In Fifteen years you have wasted and lost.....	\$424	77	8
Sixteenth Year you lose Interest Money..........	25	48	6
And, at **Five Cents per day,** you waste	18	25	
In Sixteen years you have wasted and lost	\$468	51	4
Seventeenth Year you lose Interest Money	28	11	
And, at **Five Cents per day,** you waste	18	25	
In Seventeen years you have wasted and lost ..	\$514	87	4
Eighteenth Year you lose Interest Money........	30	89	2
And, at **Five Cents per day,** you waste	18	25	
In Eighteen years you have wasted and lost ...	\$564	01	6
Nineteenth Year you lose Interest Money........	33	84	
And, at **Five Cents per day,** you waste	18	25	
In Nineteen years you have wasted and lost ...	\$616	10	6
Twentieth Year you lose Interest Money.........	36	96	6
And, at **Five Cents per day,** you waste.......	18	25	
In Twenty years you have wasted and lost.....	\$671	32	2
Twenty-first Year you lose Interest Money.......	40	27	9
And, at **Five Cents per day,** you waste	18	25	
In Twenty-one years you have wasted and lost.	\$729	85	1
Carried forward,	\$729	85	1

Amount brought forward, $729 85 1

Twenty-second Year you lose Interest Money 43 79 1
And, at **Five Cents** per day, you waste....... 18 25
In Twenty-two years you have wasted and lost. $791 89 2

Twenty-third Year you lose Interest Money 47 51 3
And, at **Five Cents** per day, you waste....... 18 25
In Twenty-three years you have wasted and lost $857 65 5

Twenty-fourth Year you lose Interest Money.... 51 45 9
And, at **Five Cents** per day, you waste....... 18 25
In Twenty-four years you have wasted and lost. $927 36 4

Twenty-fifth Year you lose Interest Money...... 55 64 1
And, at **Five Cents** per day, you waste 18 25
In Twenty-five years you have wasted and lost..$1001 25 5

Twenty-sixth Year you lose Interest Money...... 60 07 5
And, at **Five Cents** per day, you waste....... 18 25
· In Twenty-six years you have wasted and lost..$1079 58

Twenty-seventh Year you lose Interest Money... 64 77 4
And, at **Five Cents** per day, you waste....... 18 25
In Twenty-seven years you have wasted and lost$1162 60 4

Twenty-eighth Year you lose Interest Money.... 69 75 6
And, at **Five Cents** per day, you waste 18 25
In Twenty-eight years you have wasted and lost$1250 61

Twenty-ninth Year you lose Interest Money 75 03 6
And, at **Five Cents** per day, you waste 18 25
In Twenty-nine years you have wasted and lost.$1343 89 6

Thirtieth Year you lose Interest Money.......... 80 63 3
And, at **Five Cents** per day, you waste 18 25
In Thirty years you have wasted and lost......$1442 77 9

Thirty-first Year you lose Interest Money........ 86 56 6
And, at **Five Cents** per day, you waste 18 25
In Thirty-one years you have wasted and lost..$1547 59 5

Thirty-second Year you lose Interest Money 92 85 5
And, at **Five Cents** per day, you waste 18 25
In Thirty-two years you have wasted and lost..$1658 70

Thirty-third Year you lose Interest Money 99 52 2
And, at **Five Cents** per day, you waste 18 25
In Thirty-three years you have wasted and lost.$1776 47 2

Thirty-fourth Year you lose Interest Money 106 58 8
And, at **Five Cents** per day, you waste....... 18 25
In Thirty-four years you have wasted and lost. .$1901 31
Carried forward, $1901 31

Amount brought forward, $1901 31

Thirty-fifth Year you lose Interest Money 114 07 8
And, at **Five Cents per day,** you waste 18 25
In Thirty-five years you have wasted and lost.. $2033 63 8

Thirty-sixth Year you lose Interest Money.......   122 01 8
And, at **Five Cents per day,** you waste 18 25
In Thirty-six years you have wasted and lost... $2173 90 6

Thirty-seventh Year you lose Interest Money....   130 43 4
And, at **Five Cents per day,** you waste 18 25
In Thirty-seven years you have wasted and lost. $2322 59

Thirty-eighth Year you lose Interest Money 139 35 5
And, at **Five Cents per day,** you waste 18 25
In Thirty-eight years you have wasted and lost. $2480 19 5

Thirty-ninth Year you lose Interest Money 148 81 1
And, at **Five Cents per day,** you waste.......   18 25
In Thirty-nine years you have wasted and lost . $2647 25,6

Fortieth Year you lose Interest Money 158 83 5
And, at **Five Cents per day,** you waste 18 25
In Forty years you have wasted and lost $2824 34 1

Forty-first Year you lose Interest Money 169 46
And, at **Five Cents per day,** you waste 18 25
In Forty one years you have wasted and lost .. $3012 05 1

Forty-second Year you lose Interest Money 180 72 3
And, at **Five Cents per day,** you waste 18 25
In Forty-two years you have wasted and lost... $3211 02 4

Forty-third Year you lose Interest Money 192 66 1
And, at **Five Cents per day,** you waste 18 25
In Forty-three years you have wasted and lost. $3421 93 5

Forty-fourth Year you lose Interest Money 205 31 6
And, at **Five Cents per day,** you waste 18 25
In Forty-four years you have wasted and lost... $3645 50 1

Forty-fifth Year you lose Interest Money 218 73
And, at **Five Cents per day,** you waste 18 25
In Forty-five years you have wasted and lost .. $3882 48 1

Forty-sixth Year you lose Interest Money........   232 94 8
And, at **Five Cents per day,** you waste 18 25
In Forty-six years you have wasted and lost ... $4133 67 9

Forty-seventh Year you lose Interest Money 248 02
And, at **Five Cents per day,** you waste 18 25
In Forty-seven years you have wasted and lost. $4399 94 9

Carried forward, $4399 94 9

Amount brought forward, $4399 94 9
Forty-eighth Year you lose Interest Money 263 99 6
   And, at **Five Cents per day,** you waste 18 25
   In Forty-eight years you have wasted and lost . . $4682 19 5
Forty-ninth Year you lose Interest Money 280 93 1
   And, at **Five Cents per day,** you waste. 18 25
   In Forty-nine years you have wasted and lost . . $4981 37 6
Fiftieth Year you lose Interest Money 298 88 2
   And, at **Five Cents per day,** you waste. 18 25
   In Fifty years you have wasted and lost $5298 50 8

This Table forms a Basis for Computing Waste and Loss at any Daily Rate.

First Rule.—*When dissipation money averages two or more Fives per day, multiply yearly footings by as many Ones as you spend Fives.*

Example.—When a young man spends 15 cents per day to gratify his carnal appetite, how much will he waste and lose in 5 years?

Fifth year's footing (see table) $102 87 6
He spends 3 Fives, hence multiply by . . . . . .   3 Ones
                    Answer $308 62 8

Second Rule.—*When dissipation money averages 3, 7, 12, or some number of cents other than two or more Fives, first divide yearly footings by 5, then multiply the quotient by the whole number of cents spent per day.*

Dividing by 5 gives the waste and loss at an average of one cent per day.

CHRONOLOGICAL ABSTRACT OF THE INVASION OF TOBACCO.

BY H. A. DIPIERRIS, M.D.

(Translated from the French.)

1492. Discovery of America.

1518. Charles V., king of Spain, receives the first seeds of the so called panacea of the Indies.

From Spain the plant is sent to Portugal, where John Nicot, ambassador of France, gets acquainted with it.

1560. He introduces it to Catherine of Medicis, queen of France, who recommends it around the world, under the title of "Queen's Herb," as a cure for all diseases.

1586. Tobacco and the potato are introduced into England.

1600. Twelve years after Catherine of Medicis' death, tobacco, no longer protected by the queen, is prohibited in France, by severe laws, as injurious to the nation.

1604. In England, it is perceived that it causes among the people the same ravages as in France. King James I. writes a book against it, and it is banished from all Europe.

1624. Pope Urban Vincent inflicts corporal punishment and excommunication on those who make use of such a substance, as degrading to the soul as it is pernicious to the body.

1635. In France, a new ordinance prohibits its use and sale, under penalty of imprisonment and of corporal punishment.

1679. It reappears in France, protected by privilege. John Breton pays the government 250,000 francs yearly, and obtains the right of sole traffic in the panacea of the Indies.

1718. The government retakes the tobacco trade, which in 1791 brought 32,000,000 francs.

1793. The revolution gives liberty to the cultivation, to the sale, and to the use of tobacco.

1811. Napoleon I., in order to fill his coffers, retakes the right of the tobacco trade, and forms the *Régie*, the duty of which is to fabricate and sell tobacco for the benefit of the government.

1820. Congress demands the government to suppress the plague of tobacco. By the consideration of revenue which it produces, the case is successively adjourned by the government to 1826, to 1829, to 1837, to 1842, to 1852.

1852. Napoleon III., one of the greatest smokers of the time, and who died of nicotism, rebuilds the fortune of tobacco; by the example of his court, from whence come all the eccentricities and fashions, tobacco is spread around in the world.

Tobacco culture has been prohibited in Egypt by a decree of the Khedive. Those found cultivating the weed are fined $1,000 per acre.

"The cabmen of Paris are forbidden to smoke while driving."—*Christian Herald, July 12th.*

SMOKING AND CHEWING—A PARODY.

BY RUTH C. THOMPSON.

Smoking the weed by the daylight fair,
Smoking the weed by the noonday glare,
Smoking the weed by the fading light,
Smoking the weed in the solemn night—
 Oh ! what shall the harvest be ?
 Oh ! what shall the harvest be ?

CHORUS :

Sowing the seed of a poisoned brain,
Sowing and reaping both palsy and pain,
Forging the chains of **your** slavery—
Sure, ah ! sure, will the harvest be,
Sure, ah ! sure, will the harvest be.

Smoking in faces of ladies fair,
Poisoning all the ambient air,
In coaches and cars, where the ladies ride,
The room of the sick and the home of the bride—
 Oh ! what shall the harvest be ?
 Oh ! what shall the harvest be ?

Chewing the weed by the morning light,
Chewing all day and far into the night,
Defiling all places,—the high and the low,
The stairway, the carpet, the beautiful snow—
 Oh ! what shall the harvest be ?
 Oh ! what shall the harvest be ?

Smoking and chewing by day and by night,
Regardless of reason, regardless of right,
Thus filling the hearts of your friends with pain,
Resolving to quit, then yielding again—
 Oh ! what shall the harvest be ?
 Oh ! what shall the harvest be ?

CHAPTER XXVII.

THE INFALLIBLE CURE.

"My grace is sufficient for thee."

WE fully believe there is salvation from such unnatural appetites as those of tobacco smoking and chewing. If the grace of God can save from one evil habit, it can save from another, and that it has effectually done this, and preserved them in the enjoyment of their freedom, multitudes of witnesses can testify.

Dr. A. L. W. Bowers, of Winfield, Ohio, thus writes us: "Hallelujah! The days of miracles are not past with them that are in perfect love to God. I have great faith in God. God saved me from the appetite for tobacco in one minute. Glory to His holy name."

"PORTLAND, Mich., Jan. 12, 1881.

"DEAR BRO. SIMS,—When God came and undertook my case, I was an inveterate tobacco user; I chewed and smoked, and also was addicted to spirituous drink; also a tea sot; and God came in and cleansed the temple out, and made me perfectly clean inside and out, from head to foot, and from side to shoulder; glory to His great and matchless name. When God spoke, I did not stop to confer with flesh and blood; bless His name.

"I received your tracts which are opposed to this ungodliness in man; I made the best use of them I could to destroy this awful death from off our land. I distributed some of them in Portland, and set the people in trouble.

They said I was crazy.   Then I went to Baltimore, to the
conference the Church of God was holding, and I scattered
some there, and it was the means, under God, of causing
them to adopt it as one of their laws not to receive any
more ministers in their church that use tobacco.

" DANIEL HOFMAN."

Says one : " I was a great smoker : I smoked for nearly
forty years.   Again and again I resolved to give up
tobacco, but the habit was too strong for me.   I was active
in God's service and delighted to lead sinners to the
Saviour.   In seasons of religious fervor I was always at
the altar, talking to those who were seeking salvation.
One day I heard a young lady speak of a brother : 'He
came and spoke to me,' she said, 'as I knelt at the altar.
His breath made me sick, it was so foul with tobacco.' The
words came to me with wondrous power.   Perhaps people
talked just so about me.   I went to the Northport camp-
meeting.   I said to my wife, 'I am going to quit smoking.'
'You can't do it : you have tried over and over again 'for
years.' 'Well, I am going down to the grove.   I mean to
fall down on my knees, *and pray God for grace to help me.
I shant come back till I have conquered.'* I need not tell
you how long I prayed.   When I came back I handed my
old pipe—which had been my companion for years—to my
wife.   'Put that on the mantle-piece,' I said, 'I am master
now.' I not only broke off smoking, *but the love of tobacco
departed—not the least hankering remained.* Smokers and
smoking are alike indifferent to me.   I can walk among
them as the holy three walked amid the flames of the
furnace.   It is now four years since I had the fight in the
grove, and I conquered through believing prayer.   To God
be all the praise."

Rev. Zenas Osborne says : " For years, prior to my conversion to God, I believed that, 'Straight is the gate and narrow is the way which leadeth unto life.'

"The consecration to be made to receive the grace of God—and eternal life *seemed* to include everything ; *all we think—speak—or do.* To meet this demand my business relations had to be given up. I had used tobacco about twelve years ; but in making my consecration to God I left this out. It had never occurred to me that it was wicked to use it ; in fact, I had never heard or read that it was, and yet it did seem to me that preachers of the Gospel of Christ ought to be *pure.* But God, the Holy Ghost, let me see, the first time that I used it after my conversion, that it was *wrong* for me to use it. As I put the filthy stuff into my mouth, the Holy Spirit said, *What do you do that for ?* This came with such force, that I was very much startled. I replied that I used it for the dyspepsia. The Spirit said, ' You have no dyspepsia ; and if you had, tobacco would not cure, it rather creates it.' I then tried to hunt up other reasons for using it, as the Spirit of God continued to press the question, *What do you use it for ?* But all my reasons were completely upset by the clear reasoning of conscience and the Holy Ghost. I now perceived that God was trying to teach me the way of life more perfectly. He said, ' You have given yourself to me to be mine entire.' I said, ' Yea, Lord, all is thine.' ' Your body is a temple for the Holy Ghost ; you are to be temperate in all things ; nothing must enter in that defileth. Tobacco defileth it. All you possess belongs to God, your money, your time, talents—all are His, and must be used for His glory ; hence, you cannot spend your money for tobacco.' A great many ways were pointed out to me in which I could glorify God, in a proper use of what God

11

had given me, instead of an investment worse than useless.
I became satisfied that I had to abandon either the one
or the other—my tobacco, or Jesus Christ. *I could not
remain justified, and defile myself with it.* Now came the
giving-up process. I resolved to do it gradually lest I
should be made sick, for the tempter told me that would be
the result. I then threw away my box, and carried what
tobacco I had down cellar, determined not to use it but
three times each day, and thus by a gradual process work
a cure. I soon wanted a chew, down cellar I went, took
the weed; it never seemed to taste quite so good before, so
self suggested the idea of putting a *little* in my pocket; so I
put a little in my pocket, and thus I continued to do till
my tobacco was all gone, and instead of carrying it in a box
or in one pocket, I had it in nearly every pocket about me,
Oh! how mean I felt when I was brought to a realization
of my bondage to such a *filthy* habit! It had wound its
slimy folds about me so long, that I seemed to be completely within its power. But here I resolved to try the
strength and power of grace divine. I now determined to
be free—sink or swim, survive or perish; I meant to have
the victory over *this habit.* I got down before God in the
dust, told Him all about my weakness, and about this
miserable habit, and cried, 'O Lord, deliver me from this
wicked, intemperate habit;' and, blessed be God! help
came—I got the victory.

"Every band was severed. I was free. Hallelujah! and
I have ever remained free. I have not been defiled by
tobacco, only as I have come in contact with those that use
it. God took the appetite all away, so that I have never
had the least desire to return to my vomit. This victory
proved a great blessing both to soul and body. 'His
blood can make the foulest clean, His blood availed for me.'"

A Preacher's Confession.—" More than fifty years ago I learned to love tobacco, because my father did. For years I have loved it better than any food. In years past I have many times believed that, though tobacco did me some good, yet it was a great injury to my whole system, and that I was a *slave* to it. I was satisfied I did not use it to glorify God. I have many times, in twenty-five years past, tried to quit my tobacco, but did not succeed. So strong was my love and desire for it, that it seemed as though I could not live without it. The last day of December, 1870, I spent in beseeching God, with strong crying and tears, to help me. I told Him that I believed He required me to leave my tobacco, but I had used it so long, and loved it so well, that I never could quit it without His assistance. I pleaded as I rarely ever did before. The good Lord heard and answered my prayer. I have used no tobacco since, and I have had very little desire for it. I praise and thank His blessed name. I seem to have a new life.

" For more than fifty years my whole body was so filled with tobacco that I was not myself as I am now. For years I could not rest at nights. If I retired early, I could not get any sleep before the clock struck eleven, and rarely before twelve; sometimes not until three a.m. Now I retire at eight or nine o'clock, and immediately fall asleep, and awake in seven or eight hours greatly refreshed, glorifying God for His love to me.

" To two classes who read this, I wish to say a few words: (1) To those who use tobacco. Go to Jesus with your whole heart for strength, and He will hear you and give you strength to quit. You cannot do it in your own strength. (2) I beg of those who use unkind words to those who use tobacco, to do so no more, but love and pray for them. You do not know the power and strength of the love of tobacco upon the whole man. I pray God that all our bodies may be fit temples for the Holy Spirit."— *Christian Age.*

The Rev. Nathaniel Conklin says: "For thirty years or more I had been addicted to the use of tobacco. I was enamoured of it to such an extent that I would at any time have sooner gone without a meal, however inviting, than have dispensed with my tobacco after it. In other words, it had become one of the indispensables of my existence. I had become extravagant in its consumption. I used to purchase it by the pound, and scarcely ever, except when my mouth was doing duty in some other way, was it without a 'chew' in it. I was impatient of delay when necessity or politeness made me forego the pleasure of rolling the sweet morsel under my tongue. For a portion of the time I was given to the use of this quieter of the nerves, as it is sometimes called, or inspiration to thought, in both forms of its ordinary use; but smoking never had the attraction of chewing, and for some years I had ceased to use it in that form, except occasionally when I happened to meet an old friend, and we would smoke together in memory of old-time associations. I gave up smoking more particularly because I found it injurious to my throat and lungs.

"I will not say but that I essayed at different times to do the same with respect to the other habit. Time and time again I resolved to put a curb on my appetite, if I did not make a determined effort to conquer it altogether. Once I remember I limited myself to three mouthfuls a day—one after each meal, and then making the time shorter in which each mouthful should remain, encouraging myself that I would enjoy each period to the uttermost. At another time I discarded my box and its contents altogether, and then treated my resolution and my appetite at the same time by asking any I might chance to meet to furnish me with some ; but I always felt a little mean and obliged myself to explain. At the same time I felt in my heart that my resolution was mere pretence—a makeshift to quiet my conscience ; and, as the issue proved, the makeshift itself continued but for a short time. I am convinced that 'tapering off' a bad or sinful habit is not the way to conquer.

"I am very sure that had I felt then as I felt afterward, grace would have been given me to give it up. I never felt it to be a sin against the Saviour, although at times I had been troubled with misgivings, especially when I remember that holy Paul had written that all things were lawful to him, but not expedient, and he would not be brought into bondage to any. I was suspicious that I was not at perfect liberty in regard to this habit, yet consoled myself, when twinges of conscience troubled me on that point, with the boastful feeling that if it were only put forth I was possessed of power to gain the victory, not knowing then my own weakness or the bald sophistry of this whole argument both as to premise and conclusion.

"Strange to say there came to my mind a train of thought about three weeks before my deliverance, the effect of which was to lead me to reason that I had better not give it up as long as I lived. This was singular, as I had always felt that some time in the future I should give it up.

"The train of thought was perfectly quiet, and left me as quiet as it found me. I may say that I was not troubled in mind in respect to it, for it had never taken upon itself the aspect of sin. Had it so presented itself to me, no matter how great the difficulty, I should have decided to give it up forever.

"Now, I am convinced that this was the time of my ignor-

ance that God winked at; the time also, when appetite in
some measure stupefied conscience. This satisfactory determination to which I had been brought without any prompt-
ings outside of myself and entirely from a power within
and apart from myself, left me in perfect quietude. The
suggestion seemed apart from myself, because it was wholly
foreign to my previous train of thought. The only impression left upon my mind was that the experience was peculiar, and that the propriety of continuing the use of
tobacco had been decided for me and decided for my
lifetime.

"Shortly afterwards I laid in a pound of tobacco, the best
that could be purchased. About a week later I awoke one
morning, and the first thought that came to my awakened
mind after the thought of God, was to reach forth my hand
to take from the box near me my morning quantity of
tobacco. With great emphasis I was arrested. I ought—
yes, I *must* give up the use of tobacco. It was a pressure
that I could not withstand, yet it did not seem to be of the
nature of force; I had no feeling of trepidation or the
slightest feeling of unwillingness. The pressure did not
present argument or permit the making of objections, yet
it brought me at the end of three minutes that I would
rather stop using tobacco, then to the firm determination I
must stop its use then and forever. Then for the first time
I felt that my boasted strength was weakness, and under
this pressure, on the one hand, and this weakness, on the
other hand, I cried out, '*God helping me, I will!*'

"I had done my part and God did His part; rather, God
did it all, working in me to will and to do. From that
hour forth, and it is nine years last March, I have had no
desire, no appetite for tobacco. Desire and appetite have
been utterly taken away.

"For some ten days I purposely kept my box in my vest pocket, and, although it was as natural to put my hand into my pocket and take it as it was to breathe, never once during that time did I detect myself in yielding to this confirmed habit. The impulse itself was gone.

"Once I took the box out of my own will, and then it was to open it, look at its contents, and smell it. I returned it without one longing desire, one emotion of regret. From that day I have rejoiced in the liberty wherewith Christ makes His people free. Nay, more; the effect of the sudden giving up of a long-existing habit was not in the slightest measure discernible ; no restlessness of body or mind, no abstraction of thought, no inability to fix the mind for a length of time, no tendency to ill humor; which reminds me of the remark of a friend who, although strongly opposed to the use of tobacco, was glad when her husband resumed the habit, because he was so uncomfortable to live with when he tried to give it up. On the contrary, without going into particulars, the change was in all respects beneficial, without the usual drawbacks attendant upon the transition from the old to the new, from the abnormal to the normal condition.

"The way in which I was led was evidently designed to be a rebuke to my unbelief. It was in March, 1874, when this experience which has been a joy ever since, was given me. In the autumn before, as I was walking down Vesey Street in New York city, I met a college friend. Our interview was brief, for we were both in a hurry. I had time only to ask him of his welfare, to which he replied that he was very well, that his Saviour was always helping him, even to his taking away of his appetite for tobacco. This he said not only for his own sake, but more especially for mine; for he perceived, even in that little time, that my old habit still clung to me.

"After we parted, my reasoning concerning his confident statement seemed to prove to me that he was a man of emotional nature and rather inclined to enthusiasm. While I would not question his absolute sincerity, I attributed the stress of his experience very much to his own way of looking at it.

"While I knew that my Saviour could do all things for me, and while I had experience of His sympathy and help in everything pertaining to life and godliness, I did not feel any special need of His aid in this matter, as I had no desire to give up the use of tobacco. Then coming to the root of the matter, I acknowledged to myself a twinge of misgiving, that if he were the subject of a special deliverance I ought to seek the same for myself; for was not my condition one of guilt and danger as truly as his?

"These thoughts were more or less undefined and soon passed away; the only permanent impression produced was that my good brother's apprehension of the efficient cause and extent of his deliverance was an illusion.

"Afterwards when my experience confirmed me in the truth of his, I was rebuked for the slowness of my faith; remembering that with Christ all things are possible.

"This experience of my friend reminds me of one just the reverse. Soon after my settlement in the ministry, I was visited by a brother considerably my senior. As we were together putting his horse to the buggy preparatory to his departure, noticing that, as usual, I had tobacco in my mouth, he looked at me over the horse's neck and said with some impressiveness, 'Had you not better give up the use of tobacco for your children's sake if not for your own?'

"He added that for years he had been an immoderate

chewer, but had given it up, and advised me to go and do
likewise. But when he came to tell me his experience it
was anything but encouraging. He said that for two years
after he 'left off' he was most unhappy. At times he
almost feared that he would lose his mind, and even at that
day, felt the ill effect of his abstinence, and knew that his
appetite was not eradicated, but simply kept in abeyance.
I made no promise—indeed, felt deterred from doing so
because of the story of his unsuccessful conflict.

"Some twenty years from that time came my own success-
ful experience, in which I was constrained by God and by
Him sustained. During these years this brother resigned
his charge and resided at Somerville, N.J.

"Several months after my deliverance the Bible Society
met in the Reformed Church, at Bedminster, in the same
State. During intermission a circle of ministers were
gathered in front of the church. This good brother joined
the group, stationing himself in front of me. Someone
having mentioned the subject of tobacco, he pointed to me
with the remark, "Here is a brother who ought to give it
up, at all events." I replied that was not so, for I had
given it up some months since. He then turned to me
with an earnestness of manner that reminded me of the
almost desperation of his manner twenty years before, saying : 'I know how to sympathize with you.'

"I then told the story in a few words of how kindly God
had dealt with me. Instantly he responded, 'You don't
deserve any credit, then.' 'I don't take any credit; it is
all of grace,' was my quick reply. And in these words
you will find the gist of the whole of the way in which God
led me. No credit—all of grace !

"Such experiences are given to us when we, in our weakness lay hold of its strength to make known the supremacy
of God over the will of man and the beneficence of that

supremacy. We are taught the difference between being saved by works and being saved by grace.

"My good brother was kept from the use of tobacco by dogged resolution. How terribly he suffered only God knows and himself. Like Paul he was kept from outward transgression, and concerning the law, he also was blameless.

"The same principle holds good in respect to those in bondage to any worthless or vicious habit. The same is true of the soul as well as of the body. There is but one Saviour for the one and the other.

"There are thousands who are in bondage to the love—rather enslaved to the appetite—of strong drink. They resolve and resolve again to free themselves, yet find themselves bound hand and foot.

"To all such and to those enthralled by the use of tobacco or opium, or in bondage to any other evil habit, we repeat there is help for you in the keeping power of Him who is mighty—yea, Almighty, and as willing as powerful; help for all who will cry unto Him in faith. 'Will *you* do it? Will you do it *now?*'"

To all who are enslaved by the despotic power of the weed, we prescribe the following *infallible* cure :

1. Do not trifle with the habit.

2. Do not imagine that you can drop this drug by degrees. Use little as you please, and you nourish an appetite which never dies so long as fed with one morsel of aliment.

3. Use no substitutes.

4. Do not merely try to abandon tobacco. Trying and doing are two different things.

5. Abandon it now—now and forever.

6. Go to God in prayer; cry mightily to Him for the appetite to be destroyed, as well as for grace to enable you to carry out your resolution. Fully trust Him to do this

for you, and it shall be done ; yes, effectually done. *But if we walk in the light, as he is in the light, we have fellowship one with another; and the blood of Jesus Christ his Son, cleanses us from all sin.*—1 John i. 7. Hallelujah.

We have seen the effectual working of this remedy. In our pastoral labors, we have been privileged to witness a great many cases of salvation from the tobacco appetite. Their united testimony is, that they have a cleaner body, purer breath, improved health, a quicker conscience, more money, a better appetite, steadier nerves, a clearer intellect ; and, best of all, great peace with God. One old man in particular testifies that he had used it for *seventy* years, but God has completely taken from him all desire for the weed. Thank God for a *clean* salvation.

Tobacco using, though a dreadful evil, is only one of the many popular "works of the flesh," and though a man may give up his weed, unless he renounces all other sins, he is still in danger of hell. Reform, then, that is not based on a surer foundation than the mere cutting down of one of the branches of the tree of depravity, is not, and cannot be effectual. Something more radical than this must be done before the victim of the pipe or the cup can be a truly reformed man. The axe must be laid at the root of the tree. See Matt. ii. 10. There must be a mighty change wrought in his soul by the power of the Holy Ghost, saving him from the bondage of *all* depraved appetites and habits, and making him "a new creature." When this work of salvation has been wrought, the emancipated soul will neither want tobacco, strong drink, opium, snuff, cards, billiards, or any other sensual indulgence. Most assuredly he will not need to join a temperance society to keep him from drink and tobacco. *Every* chain is broken, and he has victory over the world, the flesh and the devil.

PRESS NOTICES.

From the following comments of the press the reader may form some further idea as to the character of this work :

Montreal Witness.—"The incidents and statements used are gathered from many sources, but those that will carry most conviction with them are taken from the writings of eminent physicians and medical journals, showing now what is beginning to be understood : that nations, where the use of tobacco is permitted to the young, degenerate rapidly in physical and mental power, and that paralysis, and sudden death, and numerous forms of ill-health arise from its use. . . The twelve pleas which smokers often bring up to justify themselves are answered ably and with spirit by Mr. Sims. . . We can recommend this little work to those who wish to study this subject for their own benefit, or who wish to present a short, clear, readable statement of the evils of tobacco using to their smoking friends."

Boro. of Greenwich Observer, Eng.—"America is supposed to be *par excellence* the paradise of smokers, while chewing is a habit not altogether unknown, if the stories imported from across the Atlantic contain any truth in them. The Rev. Albert Sims has written a vigorous protest against these twin evils, and if the statistics he gives are to be depended upon, there is no doubt that a vast amount of disease, as well as misery and want, are traceable to indulgence in these habits. America seems to have gone ahead of England in this particular, for while it is computed that at home some £12,000,000 are expended annually in tobacco and cigars, the consumption in the United States is put down at £50,000,000, or four times as much ! At the late New England Methodist Episcopal Conference, held in Massachusetts in 1877, Bishop Harris is reported to have said that 'the Methodist Church spends more for chewing and smoking than it gives toward converting the world."

Gospel Banner.—"It is an able work. His logic is good. He treats the question from a Christian standpoint. Those addicted to the habit of using the filthy weed should send for a copy, for he gives a sure cure, and those who will follow out his recipe will be cleansed from the appetite."

United Brethren in Christ.—"Bro. Sims is an able writer against this sin, and we are glad in God that he attacks it so earnestly and holds on to it so well. Surely the vain and utterly useless weed deserves nothing better than constant exposure and rebuke. We certainly are puzzled to think of anything that is of less use to man. Indeed, it is a real injury to him, and a disgusting, sickly, dirty thing to come in contact with. We are utterly amazed at old men continuing in the habit,—men of knowledge, men of experience and Bible light—and selling the obnoxious weed to others, and allowing their sons to grow up and start right in their steps. It pains us in our inmost soul. Oh, when will men learn to be wise! We can hardly find language to express our utter contempt of this detestable evil Every tobacco user ought to have a copy of this book ; and every opposer of tobacco ought to get copies and circulate them."

Canadian Baptist, Toronto. "The author writes very earnestly and wisely on the evil effects of nicotine upon young persons especially. He points out that the medical profession, as a whole, lends slight, if any, countenance to the formation by young men of smoking habits, and he quotes the testimony of several physicians as to the injury done to the system by nicotine. He denies that smoking is a manly practice or that it is any support to the mind in trouble or an aid to brain work, or that it assists digestion. The arguments for a Christian giving up the use of tobacco are especially deserving of attention."

Canadian Prohibitionist.—"It is addressed especially to Christian people who use tobacco, and the author endeavors to show that the habit is not only unclean, injurious to health, and a cause of waste, but is also a sin. Divine grace is presented in the infallible cure."

Our Messenger.—"We have just finished the reading of a little book, entitled, 'The Sin of Tobacco Smoking and Chewing,' by Rev. Albert Sims. The brother is an avowed enemy of the 'weed,' and a genuine hater of the habit of using it. Seemingly, for years he has been gathering testimony to secure its conviction, and perpetual banishment. We doubt not but the perusal of it will induce many to give up the filthy habit. This little work has given us a disgust for tobacco we never had before. While we do not charge *sin* upon every smoker, we at the same time do believe that the use of tobacco is a physical evil, and a moral wrong. No man can use it without injuring his influence less or more, especially with some people. No prayer-leader, class-leader, steward, local preacher, or travelling preacher, can use it and not mar his usefulness. If those in our Ministry could only see how much they are the butt of ridicule, and objects of contempt by very many of our people, they would certainly quit it."

Boyce's Saturday Anvil, Washington, D.C. "This is a well written pamphlet. It contains some of the most effective and convincing arguments against the influences of tobacco-using in all its forms that we have ever read. We are satisfied that there are many professing religion addicted to the vile habit, who would abandon it if they were convinced of its sinfulness. We believe anyone who reads this book will be convinced, and we recommend its careful perusal to all such."

The Canada Presbyterian.—"Mr. Sims has written with considerable zeal and feeling on the subject. He was evidently under the impression that he had a work to do, and he spared no effort to accomplish it. He has most industriously collected a large assortment of details illustrating the injurious effects moral and physical of tobacco in all its shapes and forms. With a most unmerciful hand he has drawn vivid pictures representing the practices of smoking and chewing in their worst aspects. . . . . The writer of the pamphlet under review commences his seventh chapter with the text, 'Thou shalt not kill,' and really we cannot question his position. We must admit that tobacco smoking to excess is a sort of slow suicide. . . . We hope that Mr. Sims' pamphlet will have a wide circulation, and that it will be the means of preventing many of the young men from acquiring pernicious habits, as well as of leading many Christian men to view the practices referred to in a new light."

Free Methodist.—"The author has put a great deal of thought in a small space. His logic is good, his style pleasing, and his arguments conclusive. He treats the question from a Christian standpoint, and makes a clear case. We are pleased to note that the remedy provided for the cure of this dreadful sin is the Blood of Christ. Some remarkable cures of both the habit and appetite are recorded. We recommend Bro. Sims' book to the careful perusal of every one who uses 'the weed' in any form, as well as to all who would be informed upon the nature and effects of this narcotic. Ministers will find the work full of thought, and really a valuable compilation. Buy and read it, and if you have a friend bound in chains of habit to this filthy god, present it to him, with a request that he read it, and a prayer that God may bless it to his enfranchisement."

Anti-Tobacco and Prohibition Tracts.

Does the Tobacco Habit Glorify God?

The Tobacco Habit: Its Sin and Cure.

Tobacco-using Parents Injure their Offspring.

Licensed Saloon.

Correspondence between the Rumseller and the Devil.

The above tracts are 25c. per 100.

ADDRESS REV. A. SIMS, UXBRIDGE, ONTARIO.

www.ingramcontent.com/pod-product-compliance
Lightning Source LLC
Chambersburg PA
CBHW031114020726
47495CB00007B/2193